Study Guide
to Accompany
Pharmacological Aspects of Nursing Care
Seventh Edition

Bonita E. Broyles

Barry S. Reiss

Mary E. Evans

Written by
Peggy S. Denning, RN, MSN, ADON

DELMAR
CENGAGE Learning·   Australia   Brazil   Canada   Mexico   Singapore   Spain   United Kingdom   United States

DELMAR
CENGAGE Learning™

Study Guide to Accompany

Pharmacological Aspects of Nursing Care, Seventh Edition

Bonita E. Broyles, Barry S. Reiss, Mary E. Evans

Written by Peggy S. Denning, RN, MSN, ADON

Vice President, Health Care Business Unit:

William Brottmiller

Director of Learning Solutions:

Matthew Kane

Acquisitions Editor:

Maureen Rosener

Product Manager:

Elizabeth Howe

Editorial Assistant:

Chelsey Iaquinta

Marketing Director:

Jennifer McAvey

Marketing Manager:

Michele McTighe

Marketing Coordinator:

Danielle Pacella

Production Director:

Carolyn Miller

Content Project Manager:

David Buddle

Art Director:

Jack Pendleton

For product information and technology assistance, contact us at
Cengage Learning Customer & Sales Support, 1-800-354-9706

For permission to use material from this text or product, submit all requests online at **cengage.com/permissions**
Further permissions questions can be emailed to
permissionrequest@cengage.com

ISBN-13: 978-1-4018-8887-9

ISBN-10: 1-4018-8887-9

Delmar Cengage Learning
5 Maxwell Drive
Clifton Park, NY 12065-2919
USA

Cengage Learning products are represented in Canada by Nelson Education, Ltd.

For your lifelong learning solutions, visit **delmar.cengage.com**

Visit our corporate website at **www.cengage.com**

Notice to the Reader

Publisher does not warrant or guarantee any of the products described herein or perform any independent analysis in connection with any of the product information contained herein. Publisher does not assume, and expressly disclaims, any obligation to obtain and include information other than that provided to it by the manufacturer. The reader is expressly warned to consider and adopt all safety precautions that might be indicated by the activities described herein and to avoid all potential hazards. By following the instructions contained herein, the reader willingly assumes all risks in connection with such instructions. The publisher makes no representations or warranties of any kind, including but not limited to, the warranties of fitness for particular purpose or merchantability, nor are any such representations implied with respect to the material set forth herein, and the publisher takes no responsibility with respect to such material. The publisher shall not be liable for any special, consequential, or exemplary damages resulting, in whole or part, from the readers' use of, or reliance upon, this material.

Printed in the United States of America
7 11 10

TABLE OF CONTENTS

PREFACE

The purpose of the *Study Guide to Accompany Pharmacological Aspects of Nursing Care,* 7th Edition is to help you learn, absorb, and retain difficult and often unfamiliar concepts in pharmacological nursing. This *Study Guide* will help reinforce major concepts as you review the central facts of each textbook chapter, and it will help you to develop the knowledge and skills you will need to succeed as a nurse in any health care setting.

Each chapter of the *Study Guide* contains learning exercises that draw on key ideas from the textbook. The activities include matching exercises, true-or-false questions, multiple choice questions, and critical thinking exercises.

CHAPTER 1 Drugs/Agents and Factors Affecting Their Action

Objectives

After reading Chapter 1 of *Pharmacological Aspects of Nursing Care*, 7th edition, the student will be able to:

■ Identify and differentiate between the basic terms of the study of pharmacology.

■ Compare and contrast the significance of the three different names given to each drug.

■ Compare and contrast the different groups of controlled substances.

■ Identify and describe the different types of drug reactions.

■ Explain the importance of understanding drug concentrations in the body.

■ Differentiate between the factors that determine drug response.

Matching

Match the following pharmacologic terms with their correct definitions.

_____ 1. pharmacokinetics

_____ 2. pharmacotherapeutics

_____ 3. pharmacogenetics

_____ 4. pharmacognosy

_____ 5. pharmacodynamics

A. study of drugs' mechanisms of action

B. study of drugs derived from herbs

C. study of absorption, distribution, metabolism, and excretion of drugs

D. study of how drugs are used in the treatment of illness

E. study of how a person responds to a drug

Match the following drugs with their major uses.

_____ 6. aspirin

_____ 7. insulin

_____ 8. contrast dye

_____ 9. penicillin

_____ 10. hepatitis vaccine

A. diagnostic drug

B. curative drug

C. preventive drug

D. symptomatic treatment drug

E. health maintenance drug

Match the following controlled substances with their proper categories (schedules).

_____ 11. Demerol

_____ 12. LSD

_____ 13. Hydrocodone

_____ 14. Librium

_____ 15. Lomotil

A. Schedule IV

B. Schedule I

C. Schedule II

D. Schedule V

E. Schedule III

True/False

Place T or F on the line before each statement.

_____ 1. Enteric coated medications should be crushed before administration in order to prevent gastric irritation.

_____ 2. The tablet is the most popular drug dosage method.

_____ 3. An ampule contains one single dose of medication for injection.

_____ 4. Controlled substances have the ability to cause physical and psychological dependence.

_____ 5. Morphine sulfate is an example of a Schedule IV drug.

_____ 6. Drugs that interact with a receptor to produce a response are known as antagonists.

_____ 7. Herbals are not regulated by the FDA.

_____ 8. Medications administered sublingually are held on the inner lining of the cheek until completely dissolved.

_____ 9. One example of the transdermal therapeutic system is fentanyl.

_____ 10. The generic name of a drug is assigned by the United States Adopted Names (USAN) Council.

Multiple Choice

Circle the best answer for each of the following questions. There is only one answer to each question.

1. The process by which a drug is carried from the absorption site to the site of action is known as
   - A. drug distribution
   - B. drug displacement
   - C. drug half-life
   - D. drug elimination

2. Paul and Walt are participants in a drug study. Both men are of the same age and are similar in body height and weight. Both men are given a test dose of the experimental drug labeled "MED A." Walt develops an adverse reaction not seen in Paul or in any other study participant. Walt's reaction is an example of
   - A. teratogenic effect
   - B. idiosyncratic effect
   - C. iatrogenic effect
   - D. carcinogenic effect

3. The herbal primarily used for the treatment of benign prostatic hypertrophy (BPH) is
   - A. gingko
   - B. echinacea
   - C. ginseng
   - D. saw palmetto

4. According to the Controlled Substance Act of 1970, controlled substances are classified into five different categories or schedules. Diazepam (Valium) falls into what category?
   - A. Schedule II
   - B. Schedule III
   - C. Schedule IV
   - D. Schedule V

5. Clinical studies performed on human subjects before marketing a product are divided into four phases. This phase involves broad clinical trials designed to evaluate drug usefulness in treating the disease for which it is claimed to be effective.
   - A. Phase I
   - B. Phase II
   - C. Phase III
   - D. Phase IV

6. Atorvastatin (Lipitor), a medication used to lower cholesterol, belongs to the following group.
   - A. curative drugs
   - B. diagnostic drugs
   - C. health maintenance drugs
   - D. preventive drugs

7. Eddie, a college freshman, has been studying for midterms for the last week. In order to stay awake for the long group "cramming sessions," Eddie has been drinking all the coffee he can get his hands on. But Eddie has a mild case of asthma requiring an occasional puff of Ventolin, which he recently took. He is now experiencing shortness of breath and tachycardia. This is an example of
   - A. drug interactions
   - B. drug elimination
   - C. drug metabolism
   - D. drug absorption

8. By the time a drug becomes available to the public, it has been given several names. Systematically derived, this term identifies the structure of the drug.
   - A. generic name
   - B. chemical name
   - C. brand name
   - D. trade name

9. One of the most popular herbals today, this is used mostly to treat memory impairment and dementia.
   A. echinacea
   B. St. John's wort
   C. gingko
   D. ginseng

10. The ability of this herbal to inhibit serotonin, dopamine, and norepinephrine reuptake in the central nervous system makes it popular for the treatment of mild to moderate depression.
    A. St. John's wort
    B. saw palmetto
    C. aloe
    D. garlic

Critical Thinking Exercises

1. Discuss the procedures necessary for safe administration of any medication given via the transdermal method. Include proper dosage, patient preparation and precautions, nursing safety precautions, and proper disposal of the patch.

   _____

   _____

   _____

   _____

   _____

2. Name and describe each component of the physician's written prescription and the significance of each. Describe the difference between the written prescription and the hospital prescription.

   _____

   _____

   _____

   _____

   _____

3. Identify and describe the factors that contribute to the individual variations of drug responses.

   _____

   _____

   _____

   _____

   _____

4. Familiarize yourself with the different drug dosage forms. Give an example of each form.

_____

_____

_____

_____

_____

5. Explain the concept of drug "half-life." Give an example.

_____

_____

_____

_____

_____

CHAPTER 2 Principles and Methods of Drug Administration

Objectives

After reading Chapter 2 of *Pharmacological Aspects of Nursing Care,* 7th edition, the student will be able to:

- Discuss the "seven rights" of medication administration.
- Identify abbreviations used in medication administration.
- Describe the steps of the nursing process and how each one relates to the administration of medications.
- Describe the different routes of medication administration.
- Demonstrate the various anatomical landmarks for administering medications by injection.

Matching

Match the following components of the nursing process with their appropriate definitions.

_____ 1. implementation	A.	gathering information to determine client's needs
_____ 2. assessment	B.	nurse determines outcomes
_____ 3. nursing diagnosis	C.	carrying out plan of care
_____ 4. evaluation	D.	identifying problem areas
_____ 5. planning	E.	establishing priorities, determining interventions, and setting outcomes

Match the following nursing abbreviations with their English meanings.

_____ 6. gtt	A.	after meals
_____ 7. KVO	B.	drop
_____ 8. IVPB	C.	intravenous piggyback
_____ 9. p.c.	D.	keep vein open
_____ 10. h.s.	E.	nasogastric tube
_____ 11. o.u.	F.	sublingually
_____ 12. NGT	G.	at bedtime
_____ 13. SL	H.	both eyes
_____ 14. a.c.	I.	before meals

True or False

Place T or F on the line before each statement.

_____ 1. The development of an anaphylactic reaction signals an immediate emergency.

_____ 2. When using a unit-dose system, open the dose before taking it to the client's bedside.

_____ 3. To remove a drug from a multi-dose vial, inject an amount of air equal to twice as much as the amount of fluid to be withdrawn.

_____ 4. One of the "seven rights" of medication administration is identifying the right client.

_____ 5. When giving an oral antacid, it is important to instruct your client not to eat or drink for 20 to 30 minutes.

_____ 6. When measuring liquid medications, hold container at eye level to pour.

_____ 7. Before administering medication to the client with a nasogastric tube, check the tube for proper placement.

_____ 8. When delivering medication via a nasogastric tube, use a 50 cc bulb syringe and push the medication through the tubing.

_____ 9. After giving medication via a nasogastric tube, it is imperative to leave the tubing unclamped.

_____ 10. Always recap the syringe after giving an intramuscular injection.

_____ 11. Subcutaneous insulin is administered at a 90-degree angle.

_____ 12. Heparin is administered in abdominal subcutaneous tissue.

_____ 13. To administer ear drops to an adult, pull the pinna up and back.

_____ 14. Leaving prescribed medications at the client's bedside is an acceptable nursing practice.

_____ 15. One reason for client noncompliance regarding drug therapy is the expense, especially among the elderly and uninsured populations.

Multiple Choice

Circle the best answer for each of the following questions. There is only one answer to each question.

1. The administration of medication via a nasogastric tube is followed by _____ of fluid.

   A. 25–75 mL
   B. 10–20 mL

   C. 30–50 mL
   D. 5–30 mL

2. For the administration of oral medications, the nurse must first

   A. check the client's identification bracelet
   B. wash his or her hands

   C. check the label on the medication three times
   D. open unit-dose packages

3. Which of the following types of oral medications should never be altered before administration?

   A. capsules
   B. tablets

   C. chewables
   D. enteric coated

4. The signs and symptoms of anaphylaxis include all of the following *except*

   A. bronchospasm
   B. hypotension

   C. hypertension
   D. laryngeal edema

5. The preferred anatomical site for the injection of 1 mL or less of a clear, nonirritating solution, such as school-age and adult immunizations, is the

   A. dorsogluteal site
   B. deltoid site

   C. ventrogluteal site
   D. vastus lateralis site

6. Site rotation is important when clients are receiving frequent intramuscular injections because

   A. drug absorption is enhanced
   B. tissue integrity is adversely effected

   C. client preference is honored
   D. lipodystrophy is prevented

7. Your hospitalized client is prescribed to receive morphine sulfate intramuscularly for pain. Your client has just returned from the post-anesthesia care unit and has an intravenous access. What action should you take when you see the intramuscular prescription for morphine sulfate?

   A. Administer it as prescribed within the frequency parameters
   B. Explain to the client that this is the prescribed route
   C. Collaborate with the health care provider to change route of administration to IV
   D. Suggest that a new nurse do the intramuscular injections "because it is good practice" for him or her

8. When an intramuscular injection of vitamin B$_{12}$ is prescribed for your hospitalized client with pernicious anemia, what should you do to decrease the pain of this injection?

    A. Collaborate with the health care provider on a prescription for the local anesthetic-eutectic mixture of lidocaine and prilocaine (EMLA)
    B. Rub the area of the injection firmly with alcohol before administering
    C. Administer the medication as quickly as possible
    D. Ask another nurse to give the injection because you don't want to hurt your client

9. Mr. Jones is to receive his enteral medications via his gastrostomy tube. He is prescribed three medications to be administered at 10:00 am. What action should the nurse take when administering these medications?

    A. Mix the medications together and flush the G-tube with normal saline after administering the medications
    B. Crush medications, mix in sterile water, and then administer the medications together
    C. Check the client's G-tube residual prior to administering the medications and discard the residual obtained
    D. Administer each medication separately and flush the G-tube with water between each one

10. You are preparing to administer an intradermal turberculin skin test to your clinic client. Which action should you take during the administration?

    A. Insert the needle with the bevel pointed downward at a 10-degree angle
    B. Insert the needle at a 15-degree angle with the bevel up
    C. Insert the medication at a 45-degree angle, ensuring that the medication is absorbed
    D. Be sure that you are using a 22-gauge, ½-inch needle

11. The posterior gluteal muscle is not a preferred site for intramuscular injections because

    A. of the risk of injecting the medication into a blood vessel
    B. of the risk of damage to the sciatic nerve
    C. of the risk of damage to the pelvic bone
    D. it is the most painful site

12. When checking a medication using the "seven rights" of medication administration, the nurse understands that this action is mandatory because

    A. it is the most effective way to prevent medication errors
    B. it is policy in all health care facilities
    C. it is the most current theory of medication administration
    D. it is the right thing to do

Critical Thinking Exercises

1. Discuss the full impact of the "seven rights" of medication administration. Define these "seven rights" and the problems that can arise if any section is overlooked.

_____

_____

_____

_____

_____

2. Describe the procedures for the administration of medications by injection, concentrating on intramuscular, intravenous, and subcutaneous. Name the injection sites, identify the anatomical landmarks, and identify when these particular sites are used.

_____

_____

_____

_____

_____

3. A useful nursing diagnosis covered in this chapter is Noncompliance R/T drug regimen. Construct a care plan based on this diagnosis.

_____

_____

_____

_____

_____

4. Explain the significance of knowing the position of the sciatic nerve when using the dorsogluteal injection site.

_____

_____

_____

_____

_____

CHAPTER 3 Intravenous Drug Therapy

Objectives

After reading Chapter 3 of *Pharmacological Aspects of Nursing Care,* 7th edition, the student will be able to:

- Describe the major reasons for the use of intravenous infusion therapy.
- Describe the complications of intravenous therapy.
- Describe the nursing interventions necessary to care for the client experiencing complications with intravenous therapy.
- Demonstrate care of a central venous access device.

Matching

Match the following terms with their correct definitions.

_____ 1. hydrostatic pressure

_____ 2. osmotic pressure

_____ 3. colloids

_____ 4. isotonic solutions

_____ 5. crystalloids

A. the amount of hydrostatic pressure needed to move particles and fluids in and out of vascular volume

B. does not alter plasma osmolality

C. solutions that raise oncotic pressure

D. the force water exerts against vessel walls

E. solutions that create osmotic pressure by dissolved ion movement

True or False

Place T or F on the line before each statement.

_____ 1. One part of preparing to deliver an intravenous medication to your client is priming the intravenous infusion equipment.

_____ 2. Intravenous infusion pumps provide a more accurate flow rate than gravity drip systems.

_____ 3. A potential complication of administering normal saline (0.9 NaCl) is hyperkalemia.

_____ 4. Plasma expanders are administered to restore circulatory hemodynamics.

_____ 5. The nurse should check for needle patency before administering intravenous medication.

_____ 6. For long-term or continuous intravenous therapy, the preferred venipuncture site is the antecubital space.

_____ 7. During intravenous therapy, the nurse's highest priority is maintaining the patency of the intravenous access.

_____ 8. Hickman catheter dressings must be changed using strict sterile technique.

_____ 9. The most common electrolytes added to intravenous fluids are potassium and sodium.

_____ 10. The most common potential complication that may occur during intravenous therapy is fluid overload.

Multiple Choice

Circle the best answer for each of the following questions. There is only one answer to each question.

1. This intravenous fluid is used to increase vascular volume and dehydrate the cells, causing them to shrink.
   A. isotonic
   B. hypertonic
   C. hypotonic
   D. hydrostatic

2. When administering medication via IV push (bolus), the nurse understands that the safest rate is

   A. 1 mL/min
   B. 0.5 mL/min
   C. 1.5 mL/min
   D. 2 mL/min

3. After administering a medication via IV push, the nurse understands that therapeutic or adverse effects will be seen

   A. within 5 to 10 minutes
   B. within 30 minutes
   C. by the end of his or her shift
   D. immediately

4. The intravenous solution that has the same osmolality as body fluids and does not alter plasma osmolality is the

   A. hypertonic solution
   B. hypotonic solution
   C. isotonic solution
   D. hydrating solution

5. Commonly used colloids include all of the following *except*

   A. albumin
   B. plasmanate
   C. Ringer's
   D. dextran

6. One of the most common electrolytes added to intravenous fluids is potassium. When the natural balance of this electrolyte is disrupted, cardiac disturbances occur that may prove fatal. Knowing this, the nurse takes special care to ensure that potassium remains within this range.

   A. 2.0–4.5 mEq/L
   B. 3.5–5.0 mEq/L
   C. 4.0–6.5 mEq/L
   D. 1.5–3.0 mEq/L

7. The client with a central venous access device (CVAD) should be monitored for an increase in temperature every

   A. 1 hour
   B. 2 hours
   C. 3 hours
   D. 4 hours

8. Tissue damage, breakdown, and sloughing that occur following infiltration of an IV delivering a toxic medication is called

   A. infiltration
   B. necrosis
   C. extravasation
   D. thrombophlebitis

Critical Thinking Exercises

1. Discuss the procedure (step by step) for initiating intravenous therapy on your client, including the correct procedure for equipment setup.

   _____

   _____

   _____

   _____

   _____

2. Explain the procedure for adding a piggyback to the main intravenous set.

   _____

   _____

   _____

   _____

   _____

3. Explain the procedure for administering an IV push (bolus) medication and the possible complications that may occur with this medication delivery method.

_____

_____

_____

_____

_____

4. Discuss the reasons for intravenous therapy.

_____

_____

_____

_____

_____

5. Discuss assessment, nursing diagnoses, plan of care, potential problems, interventions, and evaluation of intravenous therapy.

_____

_____

_____

_____

_____

6. Find the peripheral veins used in intravenous therapy. Discuss factors that are used in determining the most appropriate peripheral veins for intravenous therapy.

_____

_____

_____

_____

_____

CHAPTER 4 *Calculating Medication Dosages*

Objectives

After reading Chapter 4 of *Pharmacological Aspects of Nursing Care,* 7th edition, the student will be able to:

- State the correct formula to convert apothecary weights to metric equivalents.
- Correctly identify an improper fraction and determine which fractions are larger or smaller.
- Correctly calculate percentages, add decimals, convert pounds to kilograms, and utilize the metric system to solve mathematical problems.
- Calculate safe dosages for infants and children.
- Perform calculations needed for IV medication administration.

Matching

Match the following terms with their correct definitions.

_____ 1. ratio

_____ 2. proportion

_____ 3. gram

_____ 4. liter

A. the basic unit of volume in the metric system

B. the relationship of two quantities

C. the basic unit of weight in the metric system

D. formed by using two equal ratios

True or False

Place T or F on the line before each statement.

_____ 1. To convert a quantity in the metric system to a larger unit (e.g., milligrams to grams), move the decimal point to the left.

_____ 2. To convert a quantity in the metric system to a smaller unit (e.g., grams to milligrams), move the decimal point to the right.

_____ 3. The apothecary system is based upon grams.

_____ 4. Pediatric dosages are often calculated as milligrams per kilogram of body weight in a given period of time.

_____ 5. A nomogram is a chart that uses the height and weight of the client to estimate his or her body surface area (BSA) in square meters (m^2).

Practice Problems

1. The health care provider prescribes penicillin 500,000 units IV every six hours. You have penicillin 1,000,000 units/mL on hand. How many mL will you give?

2. The health care provider prescribes nitroglycerin gr 1/150 sublingual every five minutes times three doses. The vial in the medication cart contains nitroglycerin 0.04 mg. How many tablets will you give per dose?

3. Theophylline 100 mg po every 8 hours is prescribed. You have theophylline 400 mg/5 mL available. How much would you give?

4. The client you are caring for has a seizure disorder and needs phenytoin (Dilantin) 0.2 g po tid. The pharmacy has sent phenytoin (Dilantin) 100 mg/4 mL. How much will you give for each dose?

5. The client has a wound that needs to be irrigated with 0.25 L of sterile saline. The saline is in a one-liter bottle. How many milliliters will you use?

6. The client is to receive penicillin 2 g po now. Penicillin 500 mg/capsule is available. How many capsules will you give?

7. The health care provider asks for Drug A 12.5 mg be given to his or her client every morning. The label says Drug A 25 mg/tablet. What is the correct dose?

8. A prescription reads: K-tabs 40 meq followed by 30 mL water. The label says K-tabs 20 meq/tab. What is the correct dose?

9. An IV prescription says "add aminophylline 0.3 g to existing IV fluids." The vial is labeled aminophylline 500 mg/20 mL. How much will you add?

10. A 10-kg client needs to have 1 mg/kg of Drug B. How much does the client need over 24 hours? If the amount is to be divided into two equal doses, how much is a single dose?

11. Heparin 2500 units, administered subcutaneously, is prescribed. The vial is labeled heparin 5000 units/mL. How much will you administer?

12. A medication prescription calls for 1000 mL normal saline (NS) to be administered in five hours. The drop factor is 15. How many drops per minute will the saline be infused?

13. An infant is to receive 50 mL of 4% dextrose via water IV in four hours. At what hourly rate should the nurse set the IV infusion pump to administer this fluid?

14. 1000 mL D$_5$W are to be given at a rate of 21 gtt/min with a drop factor of 10 gtt/mL. How long will the infusion last?

15. An IV infusion of 80 mg of gentamicin in 100 mL of D$_5$W is to infuse in 30 minutes through the client's central venous access device. At what hourly rate would the nurse program the IV infusion pump to administer the gentamicin in 30 minutes?

Critical Thinking Exercises

1. Read the manufacturer's suggested dosage information found in the package insert for a selected medication. Determine if your client has been receiving a therapeutic dose.

    _____

    _____

    _____

    _____

    _____

2. What would be the first action you would take if you calculated a drug dose and found that the dose prescribed was too high for the patient?

    _____

    _____

    _____

    _____

    _____

3. What factors might the nurse need to be aware of before administering medication to a client?

    _____

    _____

    _____

    _____

    _____

4. Discuss how the following medication errors could occur: administering the wrong dose, administering an extra dose, omitting the dose, administering an unordered drug, administering by the incorrect route, and administering at the incorrect time.

    _____

    _____

    _____

    _____

    _____

CHAPTER 5 Drug Therapy for Pediatric Clients

Objectives

After reading Chapter 5 of *Pharmacological Aspects of Nursing Care*, 7th edition, the student will be able to:

- Identify factors that may result in paradoxical drug effects in children and infants.
- Discuss how children should be taught about their drug therapy.
- Correctly calculate pediatric dosages, convert pounds to kilograms, and utilize the metric system to solve medication dosage problems.
- Calculate safe dosages for infants and children.
- Perform calculations needed for IV medication administration to infants and children.

Matching

Match the following terms with their correct definitions.

_____ 1. absorption

_____ 2. biotransformation

_____ 3. distribution

_____ 4. excretion

A. the passage of a drug from its site of absorption to peripheral tissues

B. the process by which medication is broken down and enters into circulation

C. the method by which the liver inactivates a drug

D. the primary method of eliminating drugs

True or False

Place T or F on the line before each statement.

_____ 1. Infants and children may only receive oral medications.

_____ 2. Most medications are administered in milligram per pound of body weight for infants and children.

_____ 3. Infants and children should have a protected IV site.

_____ 4. For IV therapy in infants and children, needle gauges 21–27 are often used.

Multiple Choice

Circle the best answer for each of the following questions. There is only one answer to each question.

1. Drug excretion primarily occurs through the renal system. This process occurs by way of
   A. glomerular filtration
   B. passive tubular secretion
   C. active tubular reabsorption
   D. biotransformation

2. A drug is inactivated by enzymes, which promote elimination of that drug. The enzymes are produced by
   A. the spleen
   B. the liver
   C. the kidneys
   D. the pancreas

3. What is considered a "normal" adult weight for drug calculation purposes?
   A. 120 lbs.
   B. 130 lbs.
   C. 150 lbs.
   D. 100 lbs.

4. Using a nomogram that contains both height and weight data correlates fairly well to appropriate pediatric dosages. Which of the following statements is true?

    A. Using only weights provides adequate dosing information
    B. Nomograms are generally accurate only after the maturation of liver and kidney function has been attained
    C. All medications are unable to cross the blood-brain barrier
    D. Nomograms are accurate for all levels of pediatric clients

5. The preferred intramuscular injection site for infants is the

    A. gluteus maximus   C. deltoid
    B. tibialis anterior   D. vastus lateralis

6. How many cases of accidental poisoning of children are reported each year?

    A. 3–5 million   C. 5–7 million
    B. 4–6 million   D. 10 million

7. Which of the following factors is most indicative for determining the appropriate medication administration for an infant or child?

    A. the infant or child's age   C. prior experience taking medications
    B. medical history   D. developmental level

8. Infants and children are most at risk for complications related to the administration of medications due to

    A. their small size and immature renal system   C. family history of medication use
    B. their immature neurological system   D. their immature respiratory system

9. A parent's involvement when infants or children younger than age two are to receive medication should be based on

    A. the health care provider's request   C. the convenience for the nurse
    B. the principle that children should always be   D. the parent's comfort level with being actively involved
       held by the parent for medication administration

Critical Thinking Exercises

1. What factors are important to consider before administering drug therapy to children, and why are these important?

    _____

    _____

    _____

    _____

    _____

2. Discuss the two major factors that govern medication administration in children.

    _____

    _____

    _____

    _____

    _____

3. Create a visual presentation of the differences between children and adults in administration, metabolism, muscle mass, and excretion of medications.

    _____

    _____

    _____

    _____

    _____

    _____

4. Discuss the safety factors involved in administering oral medications to infants.

    _____

    _____

    _____

    _____

    _____

CHAPTER 6 Drug Therapy for Geriatric Clients

Objectives

After reading Chapter 6 of *Pharmacological Aspects of Nursing Care,* 7th edition, the student will be able to:

■ Describe anatomical and physiological factors that may result in altered drug responses in geriatric clients.

■ Compare and contrast the significance of three ways geriatric and pediatric clients react to medication.

■ Compare and contrast how different groups of medications may affect the elderly.

■ Identify medication administration principles for geriatric clients.

Matching

Match the following phases of the pharmacokinetic process with the corresponding changes that occur in the geriatric population.

_____ 1. absorption

_____ 2. distribution

_____ 3. biotransformation

_____ 4. elimination

A. glomerular filtration rate is reduced by 40–50% due to decreased renal blood flow

B. gastric emptying is slowed due to decreased muscle tone and motor activity

C. total body water is decreased; total body fat is increased

D. hepatic blood flow and enzymes are decreased

Match the following drugs with their major uses.

_____ 5. bisacodyl

_____ 6. digoxin

_____ 7. hydrochlorothiazide

_____ 8. penicillin

_____ 9. multivitamin

A. laxative

B. cardiotonic

C. diuretic

D. antibiotic

E. general vitamin supplement

True or False

Place T or F on the line before each statement.

_____ 1. Ninety-five percent of the elderly live in the community.

_____ 2. Elderly clients should receive intramuscular injections in the deltoid.

_____ 3. The best way to teach self-care skills to geriatric clients is to write the necessary steps out for them.

_____ 4. Promoting general health of geriatric clients helps to minimize adverse drug reactions.

Multiple Choice

Circle the best answer for each of the following questions. There is only one answer to each question.

1. The process that helps to transform active drugs into inactive _____ declines with age.
   A. enzymes
   B. metabolites
   C. purines
   D. biotransformation

2. Geriatric clients make up _____% of the population.
   A. 5–10
   B. 15–20
   C. 20–25
   D. 25–30

3. Elderly clients consume _____ % of all prescription drugs.
   - A. 10
   - B. 20
   - C. 30
   - D. 50

4. The absorption of drugs in the elderly
   - A. is increased due to increased bile production
   - B. is decreased due to decreased gastric acidity
   - C. is the same as in younger adults
   - D. is decreased due to greater production of hydrochloric acid

5. Older clients are at greater risk of cumulative effects of drugs because
   - A. of increased glomerular filtration rate
   - B. of decreased levels of digestive enzymes
   - C. topical absorption is faster
   - D. glomerular filtration decreases by 40–50%

6. Total body water in the elderly client is reduced, resulting in
   - A. decreased distribution of water-soluble medications
   - B. increased distribution of fat-soluble medications
   - C. decreased absorption of all medications
   - D. decreased number of intact nephrons

7. As a client ages, the blood flow to the intestines and kidneys
   - A. increases
   - B. decreases
   - C. remains the same
   - D. equalizes

8. When assessing the geriatric client who is beginning to take insulin for his Type 2 diabetes, the nurse should
   - A. demonstrate the procedure for intradermal medication administration
   - B. demonstrate how to withdraw medication from an ampule
   - C. assess for disabilities and sensory functioning
   - D. have client repeat back to you the demonstration for administering his oral insulin

Critical Thinking Exercises

1. Discuss the procedures necessary for the safe administration of any medication given to geriatric clients. Include proper dosage, patient preparation and precautions, nursing safety precautions, and proper documentation.

   _____

   _____

   _____

   _____

   _____

2. Develop a protocol or method to help a geriatric patient coordinate daily medications. Include any over-the-counter medications taken on a regular basis.

   _____

   _____

   _____

   _____

3. Identify and describe the factors that contribute to the individual variations of drug responses among elderly clients.

_____

_____

_____

_____

_____

4. Discuss which types of packaging are easily used by elderly clients.

_____

_____

_____

_____

_____

CHAPTER 7 Antimicrobial Therapy

Objectives

After reading Chapter 7 of *Pharmacological Aspects of Nursing Care*, 7th edition, the student will be able to:

- Describe how an antimicrobial agent is selected for use against a specific infectious agent.
- Compare and contrast classifications of antimicrobial and anti-infective agents.
- Compare and contrast narrow spectrum and broad spectrum anti-infective agents and what type of infection each would be appropriate for.
- Identify the steps to reconstitute medication for injection or infusion.

Matching

Match the following terms with their places in the chain of infection.

_____ 1. host

_____ 2. mode of transmission

_____ 3. reservoir

_____ 4. portal of exit

_____ 5. portal of entry

_____ 6. infectious agent

A. the disease-causing microorganism responsible for starting the infectious process

B. microorganism is removed from the reservoir through blood, feces, droplets, body fluids

C. infectious agent is passed on through blood, body fluids, feces, food, water, fecal-oral contamination

D. how the microorganism gains entry into the fomite or vector

E. the person or animal that becomes infected with the infectious agent

F. the person or animal that carries the infectious agent but may not be infected themselves

Match the following drugs with their major uses.

_____ 7. antibacterials

_____ 8. bacteriostatic

_____ 9. broad spectrum

_____ 10. bacteriocidal

_____ 11. narrow spectrum

A. destroy cell walls and prevent replication of the organism

B. inhibits growth of bacteria

C. destroys the bacteria

D. effectively works on a limited number of organisms

E. used when the identity and susceptibility to antimicrobials has not been established

True or False

Place T or F on the line before each statement.

_____ 1. The three sources of infection are bacteria, fungi, and viruses.

_____ 2. Most antifungal medications work by increasing cell wall permeability and by slowing or destroying the fungus.

_____ 3. Viruses are among the simplest living organisms.

_____ 4. Most staph infections are caused by staphylococcus aureus.

_____ 5. Linezolid is an important agent in the treatment of both VRE and MRSA.

_____ 6. Twenty-five percent of penicillin users will have an anaphylactic reaction to the medication.

_____ 7. Antacids and sodium bicarbonate may affect the absorption of oral tetracyclines.

_____ 8. Procaine penicillin is usually administered intravenously.

_____ 9. Clients receiving aminoglycosides are at risk for developing nephrotoxicity and eighth cranial nerve damage.

_____ 10. Rifampin and rifabutin cause feces, urine, saliva, tears, and soft contact lenses to become stained reddish-orange.

Multiple Choice

Circle the best answer for each of the following questions. There is only one answer to each question.

1. Bacteriocidal agents work by killing the microbes responsible for an infection. Which of the following groups are bacteriocidal agents?

    A. urinary tract anti-infectives
    B. cephalosporins
    C. clarithromycin
    D. tetracyclines

2. Bacteriostatic agents work by inhibiting the growth of microorganisms. The classifications of these medications include

    A. tetracyclines and macrolides
    B. azithromycin and doxycycline
    C. minocycline and erythromycin
    D. neomycin and pyridium

3. Antimicrobial agents may cause adverse effects on the client. Which of the following is an adverse effect specific to aminoglycosides?

    A. nausea and vomiting
    B. hepatotoxicity
    C. diarrhea and abdominal pain
    D. ototoxicity

4. The adverse effect associated with vancomycin is

    A. hepatotoxicity
    B. nephrotoxicity
    C. ototoxicity
    D. gastrointestinal toxicity

5. One of the drawbacks of using broad-spectrum antibiotics is the impact on the body's beneficial microorganisms. When normal flora are also killed, this is termed

    A. nosocomial infection
    B. synergistic infection
    C. superinfection
    D. iotragenic reaction

6. This broad-spectrum agent has an adverse effect of photosensitivity and may damage tooth enamel.

    A. metronadazole
    B. azithromycin
    C. norfloxacin
    D. tetracycline

7. This medication is frequently used to treat fungal infections caused by protozoa and severe anaerobic infections.

    A. clindamycin
    B. tetracycline
    C. metronidazole
    D. penicillin

8. A tick bite from spirochete Borrelia burgdorferi causes this disease.

    A. rheumatoid arthritis
    B. tuberculosis
    C. Lyme disease
    D. Rocky Mountain spotted fever

9. One recognized treatment for tuberculosis is a combined treatment of antitubercular medications, including

    A. ceftazidime and tetracycline
    B. INH and rifampin
    C. penicillin and amoxicillin
    D. gentamycin and vancomycin

10. The antiviral agent used to treat HIV infections is

    A. vidarabine
    B. ribavirin
    C. zidovudine
    D. amantadine

Critical Thinking Exercises

1. Discuss the procedures necessary for the safe administration of antimicrobial medications given to clients.

   _____

   _____

   _____

   _____

   _____

2. Develop a method to help a client coordinate daily medications. Include any over-the-counter medications taken on a regular basis and any precautions of which the client must be aware.

   _____

   _____

   _____

   _____

   _____

3. Present a teaching plan for clients receiving antimicrobial agents.

   _____

   _____

   _____

   _____

   _____

4. Discuss why chloramphenicol is no longer a first-line medication to treat infectious disorders.

   _____

   _____

   _____

   _____

   _____

CHAPTER 8 Antiparasitic Drug Therapy

Objectives

After reading Chapter 8 of *Pharmacological Aspects of Nursing Care,* 7th edition, the student will be able to:

- Describe how an antiparasitic agent is selected for use against a specific parasite.
- Discuss how humans may contract a parasite.
- Discuss the steps to prevent reinfestation of parasites.

Matching

Match the following terms with their correct definitions.

_____ 1. pediculosis

_____ 2. helminthiasis

_____ 3. amebiasis

_____ 4. malaria

_____ 5. parasites

A. parasitic disease characterized by invasion of the large bowel by protozoa

B. infestation of parasitic worms

C. infestation of lice

D. protozoa infection characterized by recurrent chills, fever, and prostration

E. may be contracted by person-to-person contact, insects, direct contact with parasites or bed linens, or contaminated food or water

True or False

Place T or F on the line before each statement.

_____ 1. Parasitic infections are classified as dermatological, gastrointestinal, or systemic.

_____ 2. Malaria is caused by protozoal parasites of the genus Plasmodium.

_____ 3. Drug therapy for malaria should prevent exacerbation and suppress symptoms during the acute symptomatic stage.

_____ 4. Mefloquine has many more adverse effects than quinine.

_____ 5. Primaquine phosphate and chloroquine are used concurrently to prevent malarial attacks.

Multiple Choice

Circle the best answer for each of the following questions. There is only one answer to each question.

1. Quinine sulfate was a commonly used antimalarial drug. Currently, quinine is used for its analgesic and skeletal muscle relaxant effects. Which of the following conditions is quinine used for?

   A. arthritis
   B. influenza
   C. leprosy
   D. amebiasis infections

2. One of the safest and most effective antimalarial agents is

   A. atovaquine
   B. chloroquine
   C. metronidazole
   D. mebendazole

3. Which of these antimalarial medications is/are commonly used to treat rheumatoid arthritis and discoid lupus erythematosus?

   A. lindane
   B. quinine sulfate
   C. fefloquine hydrochloride
   D. chloroquine

4. Which of the following medications was approved by the FDA in 1992 but was not marketed until 1998, due to allegations that it caused prolonged QT intervals?

    A. quinine

    B. chloroquine

    C. halofantrine hydrochloride

    D. pyrimethamine

5. Amebiasis is commonly treated with which of the following medications?

    A. metronidazole (Flagyl)

    B. paromomycin (Humatin)

    C. halofantrine (Halfan)

    D. hydroxychloroquine (Plaquenil)

6. Pneumocystis carinii frequently causes pneumonia in AIDS clients. Which of the following medications is effective against *Pneumocystis carinii*?

    A. atovaquone (Mepron)

    B. paramomycin (Humatin)

    C. eflornithine (Ornidyl)

    D. emetine hydrochloride

7. Your client has been diagnosed with African trypanosomiasis (sleeping sickness). What would be the ordered treatment?

    A. ivermectin 150–200 mcg × one dose orally

    B. praziquantel 20 mg/kg orally in three doses × one day

    C. chloroquine 1 g daily × two days, followed by 0.5 g × 14–21 days

    D. eflornithine hydrochloride 100 mg/kg IV every six hours × 14 days

8. The most commonly diagnosed form of helminthiasis is found in humans, evidenced by

    A. red, pruritic skin

    B. serous drainage

    C. infestation with parasitic worms

    D. scabies

9. Pyrantel parmoate (Antiminth, Combantrin) is the treatment of choice for

    A. scabies

    B. *Pneumocystis carinii*

    C. roundworms and pinworms

    D. pediculosis

10. An antiprotozoal that is also active against *Pneumocystic carinii* is

    A. atovaquone (Mepron)

    B. crotamiton

    C. permethrin

    D. malathion

Critical Thinking Exercises

1. Discuss the procedures necessary for the safe administration of antiparasitic medications for clients and the major uses, side effects, contraindications, and routes of administration of each classification.

    _____

    _____

    _____

    _____

    _____

2. Describe each parasitic infestation and the presenting signs and symptoms of each type.

    _____

    _____

    _____

    _____

    _____

3. Discuss critical laboratory values that need to be monitored for clients receiving antimalarials and antihelmintics.

_____

_____

_____

_____

_____

4. Discuss and compare nursing interventions for clients diagnosed with malaria, parasites, and helminthes.

_____

_____

_____

_____

_____

CHAPTER 9 Antiseptics and Disinfectants

Objectives

After reading Chapter 9 of *Pharmacological Aspects of Nursing Care,* 7th edition, the student will be able to:

■ Discuss the classifications of antiseptics and disinfectants, and be able to give an example of each.

■ Discuss the differences between antiseptics, disinfectants, and germicides.

■ Discuss nursing interventions and precautions for antiseptic, disinfectant, and germicide administration.

Matching

Match the following terms with their correct definitions.

_____ 1. disinfectant

_____ 2. antiseptic

_____ 3. germicide

_____ 4. prophylaxis

_____ 5. antipruretic

A. preventative

B. kills or inhibits growth of microorganisms

C. inhibits itching

D. destroys pathogenic microorganisms and helps to prevent infection

E. capable of destroying microorganisms

True or False

Place T or F on the line before each statement.

_____ 1. The most effective way to prevent the transmission of microorganisms is through the use of antibacterial scrubs and gels.

_____ 2. Benzoyl peroxide is the most effective treatment for acne.

_____ 3. Hydrogen peroxide must be mixed immediately before using, since stored solutions rapidly lose their effectiveness.

_____ 4. Dakin's solution may cause delayed wound healing and interfere with the clotting process.

_____ 5. The use of gloves decreases the need for hand washing.

_____ 6. Antiseptics and disinfectants increase cell wall permeability by denaturing the proteins and oxidizing cellular components.

_____ 7. Cresol is three times as potent as phenol.

_____ 8. Resourcinol is half as effective as phenol.

Multiple Choice

Circle the best answer for each of the following questions. There is only one answer to each question.

1. Which of the following bacteriostatic agents can cause intramyelinic edema, damaged nerves, and may cause seizures and encephalopathy?

   A. ethyl alcohol

   B. isopropyl alcohol

   C. formaldehyde

   D. hexachlorophene

2. Administration of this alcohol/aldehyde can cause vasodilation and increase bleeding at incision or injection sites.

   A. isopropyl alcohol

   B. ethyl alcohol

   C. formaldehyde

   D. glutaraldehyde

3. This agent is used to disinfect surgical instruments and other inanimate objects.

   A. formaldehyde
   B. hexachlorophene
   C. glutaraldehyde
   D. iodine

4. Which one of the following acids may be absorbed through the skin and can cause toxicity?

   A. salicylic acid
   B. boric acid
   C. hippuric acid
   D. nalidixic acid

5. This medication is used to treat urinary tract infections, and it also works well on infections caused by E. coli and some strains of Proteus.

   A. salicylic acid
   B. nalidixic acid
   C. acetylsalicylic acid
   D. benzalkonium chloride

6. A gas at room temperature, and unstable in aqueous solutions, this agent is a potent germicide.

   A. mercury
   B. benzalkonium chloride
   C. chlorine
   D. benzoic acid

7. Your client has burns on the face, both arms, and the chest. This germicidal is a compound used to help prevent infection but rapidly becomes inactivated by body fluids.

   A. chlorine
   B. mercury
   C. benzalkonium chloride
   D. silver sulfadiazine

8. Effective against both gram-negative and gram-positive organisms, this agent is a preoperative skin scrub for the client and is also used as an oral rinse to prevent gingivitis.

   A. chlorhexidine
   B. iodine
   C. benzoic acid
   D. resorcinol

9. Studies have shown that bacterial counts are lower on persons using _____ as an antimicrobial agent to wash their hands.

   A. 2–4 mL
   B. 3–5 mL
   C. 5–7 mL
   D. 1–3 mL

Critical Thinking Exercises

1. Discuss the nursing process for using antiseptics and disinfectants.

   _____

   _____

   _____

   _____

2. Review material safety data sheets for antiseptics, disinfectants, and germicides, and create a visual presentation.

   _____

   _____

   _____

   _____

   _____

3. Make a master list of antiseptics, disinfectants, and germicides for future use.

_____

_____

_____

_____

_____

CHAPTER 10 Analgesics and Antipyretics

Objectives

After reading Chapter 10 of *Pharmacological Aspects of Nursing Care,* 7th edition, the student will be able to:

■ Identify the classes, therapeutic actions, and adverse effects of analgesics and antipyretics.

■ Discuss how to determine which medication is appropriate for pain or fever.

■ Discuss the gate control theory of pain.

■ Discuss nursing interventions associated with pain control and fever.

Matching

Match the following terms with their correct definitions.

_____ 1. pain threshold

_____ 2. analgesic

_____ 3. pain tolerance

_____ 4. gate control theory of pain

_____ 5. neurotransmitters

_____ 6. anticoagulant

A. massaging or rubbing a painful area interrupts pain impulses before they are transmitted to higher brain centers where pain is interpreted

B. the amount of pain an individual can withstand without disrupting normal functions or requiring analgesic therapy

C. relieves pain without causing a loss of consciousness

D. the level of stimulus resulting in the perception of pain

E. chemical messengers

F. causes blood to become thinner

True or False

Place T or F on the line before each statement.

_____ 1. Ergotamine tartrate, methylsergide maleate, and rizatriptan are medications used to treat chronic pain.

_____ 2. All opioid analgesics must be preservative free for epidural or intrathecal administration.

_____ 3. Clients receiving opioid analgesics should drink 2400 to 3000 mL of fluid per day, unless contraindicated.

_____ 4. The greatest difficulty in treating terminally ill clients is staff attitude toward administering large doses of scheduled medications, resulting in unrelieved pain.

_____ 5. Patient-controlled analgesia increase the client's dependence upon pain medication.

_____ 6. Alternating acetaminophen and aspirin in children produces favorable antipyretic results.

Multiple Choice

Circle the best answer for each of the following questions. There is only one answer to each question.

1. The preferred method of administering analgesics for acute pain in the hospital setting is
   A. intravenously
   B. subcutaneously
   C. intramuscularly
   D. orally

2. Potentiation is a term that means
   A. A medication's effects will be increased when given with another medication.
   B. Two medications work together to provide therapeutic results.
   C. The central nervous system will be depressed.
   D. A medication's effects will be decreased when given with a second medication.

3. The most common adverse effect of opioid analgesics is

   A. nausea　　　　　　　　　　C. vomiting

   B. constipation　　　　　　　　D. diarrhea

4. The most commonly abused opioid narcotic is

   A. hydrocodone　　　　　　　　C. heroin

   B. hydromorphone HCl　　　　　D. codeine

5. An opioid antagonist is given to reverse respiratory depression caused by narcotic administration. Which antagonist would commonly be prescribed?

   A. naloxone HCl　　　　　　　　C. oxycodone

   B. hydromorphone　　　　　　　D. hydromorphone HCl

6. This medication is the most widely used analgesic/antipyretic.

   A. pentazocine hydrochloride　　C. acetylsalicyclic acid

   B. acetaminophen　　　　　　　D. salicylic acid

7. One consideration when deciding if a client should have a PCA pump is

   A. the client's age　　　　　　　C. the client's level of consciousness

   B. the client's developmental level　D. the client's ability to understand and follow directions

8. Acute pain is defined as

   A. a duration lasting less than six months with one or more episodes of exacerbation

   B. pain lasting two weeks or more

   C. recurrent pain lasting six months or more

   D. pain unrelieved by the usual methods

   E. none of the above

9. According to Joint Council on Accreditation of Healthcare Organizations (JCAHO) guidelines, a client in a hospital setting should be assessed for pain how often?

   A. every hour　　　　　　　　　C. every four hours

   B. every two hours　　　　　　　D. when the client complains of pain

10. Clients receiving fentanyl citrate for acute pain should be monitored for

    A. nausea　　　　　　　　　　C. urticaria

    B. vomiting　　　　　　　　　　D. respiratory depression

Critical Thinking Exercises

1. Discuss the procedures necessary for the safe administration of opioid medications, as well as the necessary documentation.

   _____

   _____

   _____

   _____

   _____

2. Create a detailed list of each medication classification and the major uses, adverse effects, contraindications, and routes of administration of each medication.

_____

_____

_____

_____

_____

3. Practice programming an IV pump and a patient-controlled analgesia pump, unless restricted by your state board of nursing regulations.

_____

_____

_____

_____

_____

CHAPTER 11 *Anesthetics*

Objectives

After reading Chapter 11 of *Pharmacological Aspects of Nursing Care,* 7th edition, the student will be able to:

- Discuss the classifications of anesthetics, their therapeutic actions, and the adverse effects of each type.
- Discuss the characteristics of the four stages of general anesthesia.
- Discuss how to determine which medication is appropriate for specific types of surgery.
- Discuss nursing interventions associated with pain control.

Matching

Match the following terms with their correct definitions.

_____ 1. sedative-hypnotic

_____ 2. anesthetics

_____ 3. general anesthesia

_____ 4. regional anesthesia

_____ 5. spinal anesthesia

A. anesthetic is injected into the subarachnoid or epidural space surrounding the spinal cord

B. agents that interfere with nerve conduction and cause diminished pain and sensation

C. partial or complete loss of consciousness

D. provides sedation and relieves pre-op anxiety, but does not depress respirations

E. blocks nerves only in a specific area and does not cause loss of consciousness

True or False

Place T or F on the line before each statement.

_____ 1. Anesthetics are agents that interfere with nerve conduction.

_____ 2. Propofol (Diprivan) may be administered intravenously and is compatible with blood, serum, and plasma.

_____ 3. Most clients develop tolerance to anesthetics and analgesics.

_____ 4. Anticholinergic medications increase diaphoresis and salivation.

_____ 5. Succinylcholine chloride and tubocurarine chloride provide permanent skeletal muscle relaxation.

Multiple Choice

Circle the best answer for each of the following questions. There is only one answer to each question.

1. The adverse effect associated with general anesthesia that has been almost completely eliminated due to the use of balanced anesthesia is
   A. analgesia
   B. chills
   C. hypotension
   D. nausea and vomiting

2. Respiratory collapse followed by complete circulatory collapse occurs during this toxic stage of anesthesia.
   A. stage I—analgesia
   B. stage II—delirium
   C. stage III—surgical anesthesia
   D. stage IV—medullary paralysis

3. Thiopental sodium, ketamine, methohexital sodium, and thiamylal sodium are examples of
   A. antianxiety agents
   B. ultrashort-acting barbiturates
   C. sedative-hypnotics
   D. anticholinergics

4. Which of the following benzodiazepine medications induces anesthesia within 1.5 to 2.5 minutes, depending on whether a narcotic drug has been administered at the same time?

A. etomidate

B. pentobarbital

C. promethazine

D. midazolam hydrochloride

5. Malignant hyperthermia may occur when this anesthetic is used intraoperatively or during times of extreme stress.

A. dantrolene

B. lidocaine

C. succinylcholine

D. buprivacaine hydrochloride

6. Regional anesthesia selection should be based primarily upon

A. client preference

B. the area to be anesthetized

C. the cost of the agent

D. health care provider's prior experience with the drug

7. The nurse must assess the postoperative client frequently during the immediate postoperative period in order to protect the safety of the client. What is the nurse looking for?

A. return of reflexes

B. reactivity of the pupils

C. anxiety or behavioral changes

D. complete recovery from anesthesia

8. Which of the following medications is used concurrently with midazolam as a premedication for surgical anesthesia?

A. promethazine

B. droperidol

C. fentanyl citrate

D. diazepam

9. Promethazine hydrochloride is frequently used as a sedative-hypnotic and may be combined with a reduced dose of opioid analgesic. Of what side effect should the nurses be especially aware?

A. The medication should only be injected into large veins.

B. It may cause discoloration of the urine, to pink or reddish brown.

C. It may cause flushing.

D. Protect from light to prevent precipitation.

10. All of the following nursing diagnoses would be appropriate for the preoperative client, except

A. risk of injury or falls related to CNS effects of preanesthetic agents

B. fear or anxiety related to the unknown risks of surgery and new experience

C. deficient knowledge related to preanesthetic agents and safety precautions

D. social isolation related to protective isolation

Critical Thinking Exercises

1. Discuss preoperative information that is needed prior to the client undergoing anesthesia, as well as the significance of each piece of data.

_____

_____

_____

_____

_____

2. Discuss the actions and uses of the major classes of anesthetic agents, along with their mechanisms of action, and provide an example of each.

_____

_____

_____

_____

_____

3. Discuss complications that may occur with anesthetics.

_____

_____

_____

_____

_____

CHAPTER 12 Anti-inflammatory Agents

Objectives

After reading Chapter 12 of *Pharmacological Aspects of Nursing Care,* 7th edition, the student will be able to:

■ Discuss the types, therapeutic actions, and adverse effects of anti-inflammatory medications.

■ Discuss how nonsteroidal anti-inflammatory drugs (NSAIDs) work to relieve inflammation.

■ Discuss the characteristics and differences of mineralocorticoids and glucocorticoids.

■ Apply the nursing process to patient teaching (i.e., what would you teach the client about NSAIDs and steroids?).

■ Discuss nursing interventions associated with pain control and fever.

Matching

Match the following terms with their correct definitions.

_____ 1. inflammation

_____ 2. salicylates

_____ 3. nonsteroidal anti-inflammatory drugs

_____ 4. gastric distress and occult bleeding

_____ 5. corticosteroids

_____ 6. mineralocorticoids

_____ 7. aspirin

A. a group of synthetic medications that works by inhibiting prostaglandins

B. made in the adrenal cortex and acts on the distal tubules of the kidney

C. dramatically reduces inflammation but suppresses the body's immune response

D. the most potent prostaglandin inhibitor and anti-inflammatory

E. the most common side effects of NSAIDs

F. may be used for systemic inflammation

G. vascular and delayed cellular response to invaders or injury

True/False

Place T or F on the line before each statement.

_____ 1. NSAIDs generally do not have any side effects.

_____ 2. The generic name for aspirin is acetaminophen.

_____ 3. Mineralocorticoids and corticosteroids have the same mechanism of action.

_____ 4. Ketorolac tromethamine provides opiate-level pain relief.

_____ 5. Gold therapy must be administered intramuscularly.

_____ 6. Hydroxychloroquine may cause irreversible retinal damage.

_____ 7. Indomethacin is safe to administer to clients with aspirin allergies.

_____ 8. Stomatitis and dermatitis are the most common complications among clients receiving gold therapy.

Multiple Choice

Circle the best answer for each of the following questions. There is only one answer to each question.

1. How is aspirin usually administered when used as an anti-inflammatory agent?

   A. once a day
   B. in divided doses
   C. on an empty stomach
   D. before bed

2. Clients who have allergies to aspirin usually have those same allergies associated with

   A. acetaminophen   C. antirheumatic agents
   B. corticosteroids   D. nonsteroidal anti-inflammatory drugs

3. The most common adverse effect of anti-inflammatory agents is

   A. gastrointestinal distress   C. neurotoxicity
   B. constipation   D. abdominal pain

4. The maximum dose of ibuprofen is ____ mg.

   A. 2400   C. 1600
   B. 3200   D. 2000

5. Anti-inflammatory effects usually are not evident until ____ week(s) after initiating therapy.

   A. one   C. three
   B. two   D. four

6. The least potent corticosteroid is

   A. dexamethasone   C. hydrocortisone
   B. prednisone   D. methylprednisolone

7. The nurse must assess the client frequently to protect the safety of the client. Which of the following medications may exacerbate epilepsy and psychiatric disturbances?

   A. misoprostol   C. pyroxidine
   B. phenylbutazone   D. indomethacin

8. Local applications of corticosteroids may cause suppression of the

   A. parasympathetic system   C. hypothalamic-pituitary-adrenal system
   B. sympathetic system   D. autonomic nervous system

Critical Thinking Exercises

1. Research the signs and symptoms of salicylate toxicity.

   _____

   _____

   _____

   _____

2. Create a visual presentation of the major classes of anti-inflammatory agents, along with their uses and mechanisms of action, and provide an example of each.

   _____

   _____

   _____

   _____

3. Discuss complications of corticosteroid and mineralocorticoid use. Give an example of each.

    _____

    _____

    _____

    _____

    _____

4. Describe the effects of long-term steroid use on the body.

    _____

    _____

    _____

    _____

    _____

CHAPTER 13 Agents Used to Treat Hyperuricemia and Gout

Objectives

After reading Chapter 13 of *Pharmacological Aspects of Nursing Care,* 7th edition, the student will be able to:

- Discuss the types, therapeutic actions, and adverse effects of medications used to treat hyperuricemia and gout.
- Apply the nursing process to patient teaching (i.e., what would you teach the client about gout and hyperuricemia?).
- Discuss nursing interventions and rationales associated with the administration of allopurinol (Zyloprim) and probenecid (Benemid).

Matching

Match the following terms with their correct definitions.

___ 1. gout		A. formed by the breakdown of protein
___ 2. tophi		B. a metabolic disease caused by hyperuricemia
___ 3. Uric acid		C. increases the urinary excretion of uric acid
___ 4. metatarsophalangeal joint		D. the accumulation of uric acid crystals in tissues and joints
___ 5. uricosuric agents		E. the most common area affected by gout
___ 6. purines		F. have been shown to increase the incidence of gout

True or False

Place T or F on the line before each statement.

___ 1. Probenecid's uricosuric activity may be decreased by administering salicylates at the same time.

___ 2. The most commonly used drug to treat gout is allopurinol.

___ 3. Probenecid (Benemid), allopurinol (Zyloprim), and azathioprine (Imuran) have the same mechanism of action.

___ 4. Indomethacin (Indocin) should not be used during an acute attack.

___ 5. Nonsteroidal drugs are not used for the treatment of gout.

Multiple Choice

Circle the best answer for each of the following questions. There is only one answer to each question.

1. How is colchicine usually administered during an acute gout attack?
   A. once a day
   B. every one to two hours
   C. on an empty stomach
   D. every eight hours

2. Clients taking colchicines should be monitored for
   A. tinnitus
   B. leukopenia
   C. anaphylactic reactions
   D. ototoxicity

3. The most common adverse effects of anti-gout medications are
   A. gastrointestinal distress and constipation
   B. tachycardia and bradypnea
   C. turns the urine orange and decreases pain
   D. gastrointestinal distress and diarrhea

4. Joint pain and swelling usually subside within_____ hours of the administration of colchicines.
   A. 10
   B. 12
   C. 6
   D. 24

5. Your client is prescribed colchicines and asks you how effective this drug is for people with gouty arthritis. Your best response would be

   A. "Colchicine is successful in treating the pain of gout in about 50% of clients."
   B. "Colchicine is successful in relieving acute gouty attacks in about 90% of clients."
   C. "We really don't have any statistics on this drug, but your doctor prescribes it to all of his patients with arthritis."
   D. "It isn't as effective as nonsteroidal anti-inflammatory drugs, but this is what your doctor prefers."

6. The nurse must assess the client frequently to confirm that the client is not experiencing an adverse reaction to a medication. Which of the following medications requires monitoring of complete blood count, uric acid levels, and hepatic and renal functions?

   A. allopurinol (Zyloprim)
   B. probenecid (Benemid)
   C. colchicine
   D. indomethacin (Indocin)

7. Drug-drug interactions with colchicines occur with the concurrent use of which of the following medications?

   A. cyclosporine
   B. ibuprofen
   C. acetaminophen
   D. sympatholytic agents

Critical Thinking Exercises

1. Discuss the signs and symptoms of colchicine toxicity.

2. Research the major classes of anti-gout agents, along with their uses and mechanisms of action, and provide an example of each.

3. Research and describe the effects of long-term colchicine and probenecid (Benemid) use on the body.

CHAPTER 14 Antihistamines and Nasal Decongestants

Objectives

After reading Chapter 14 of *Pharmacological Aspects of Nursing Care,* 7th edition, the student will be able to:

- Describe the signs and symptoms of the common cold and allergic rhinitis.
- List the common adverse effects of antihistamines.
- Provide the definition of allergic rhinitis.
- Discuss the major types, therapeutic actions, and adverse effects of antihistamines and nasal decongestants.
- Discuss the interactions between antihistamines and other medications.
- Describe nursing interventions associated with the administration of antihistamines and nasal decongestants.

Matching

Match the following terms with their correct definitions.

_____ 1. rhinitis

_____ 2. decongestants

_____ 3. phenylproponolamine HCl

_____ 4. budesonide

_____ 5. antihistamines

_____ 6. aspirin

A. the FDA ordered the removal of this from all drug products in the year 2000

B. this medication should be stored with the valve facing downward

C. another name for the common cold

D. this medication is used primarily for the treatment of allergic rhinitis

E. constrict nasal blood vessels by acting on alpha-adrenergic nerve receptors

F. the use of this medication may cause Reye's syndrome in children

True or False

Place T or F on the line before each statement.

_____ 1. Antihistamines are commonly used for nasal allergies.

_____ 2. Meclizine may be used in children under 12 years of age.

_____ 3. Pseudoephedrine HCl may be safely administered to clients who are pregnant or planning to become pregnant.

_____ 4. Rebound nasal congestion occurs in clients who are unable to use prescription antihistamines.

_____ 5. Antihistamines' mechanism of action is to decrease histamine release.

_____ 6. Drowsiness, dry mouth, and fatigue may decrease with continued use of cetirizine HCl.

_____ 7. Erythromycin may be safely administered concurrently with fexofenadine.

Multiple Choice

Circle the best answer for each of the following questions. There is only one answer to each question.

1. Which of the following medications may be used as a sedative, antiemetic, and adjunct to analgesics?

   A. triprolidine HCl

   B. propylhexedrine

   C. promethazine HCl

   D. pseudoephedrine

2. Allergic rhinitis is defined as

   A. an immunological response caused by allergens contacting the nasal mucosa

   B. a series of immunological responses

   C. a condition caused by a virus

   D. pharyngeal irritation

3. Which of the following antihistamines may cause cardiac arrhythmias or death when administered with erythromycin, ketoconazole (Nizoral), or itraconazole (Sporanox)

   A. cetirizine

   B. pseudoephedrine

   C. terfenadine

   D. loratidine

4. One complication of therapy with dimenhydrinate HCl is

   A. cardiac toxicity

   B. somnolence

   C. anemia

   D. may mask ototoxicity of other drugs

5. Topical decongestants should be given to children ____minutes prior to meals.

   A. 15

   B. 30

   C. 20

   D. 45

6. Which of the following medications does not exert antihistamine, bronchodilator, or anti-inflammatory activities?

   A. fexofenadine

   B. diphenhydramine HCl

   C. fluticasone HCl

   D. l-desoxyephedrine

7. Decongestants and antihistamines should be used with caution in clients with which of the following conditions?

   A. narrow-angle glaucoma

   B. respiratory infections

   C. sinusitis

   D. allergic rhinitis

8. Which of the following medications may be administered safely to clients with hypertension, heart disease, diabetes, and hyperthyroidism?

   A. ephedrine

   B. nasal decongestants

   C. diphenhydramine HCl

   D. antihistamines

Critical Thinking Exercises

1. List major types of antihistamines and nasal decongestants, and describe their effects and contraindications.

   _____

   _____

   _____

   _____

   _____

2. Create a teaching plan for your client taking antihistamine medications, including interventions and ways to maintain client safety.

   _____

   _____

   _____

   _____

   _____

3. Provide information on how coryza and allergic rhinitis are classified and diagnosed.

_____

_____

_____

_____

_____

CHAPTER 15 Expectorant and Antitussive Agents

Objectives

After reading Chapter 15 of *Pharmacological Aspects of Nursing Care,* 7th edition, the student will be able to:

- List the common adverse effects of expectorants and antitussives.
- Discuss the major types, therapeutic actions, and adverse effects of expectorants and antitussive agents.
- Discuss the interactions between antitussives and other medications.
- Discuss nursing interventions associated with the administration of expectorants and antitussive agents.

Matching

Match the following terms with their correct definitions.

_____ 1. expectorant

_____ 2. guaifenesin

_____ 3. antitussive

A. the most popular expectorant tolerated by most clients

B. decreases the frequency of involuntary cough

C. decreases the viscosity of sputum and facilitates expectoration

True or False

Place T or F on the line before each statement.

_____ 1. Guaifenesin is commonly used for nasal congestion.

_____ 2. Potassium iodide may be safely used in children under 12 years of age.

_____ 3. Benzonatate is a derivative of procaine.

Multiple Choice

Circle the best answer for each of the following questions. There is only one answer to each question.

1. Clients with heart failure who receive forced fluids may become overhydrated. You would expect to see all of the following signs and symptoms *except*

   A. moist respiration
   B. edema
   C. full, bounding pulse
   D. hypotension

2. Which clients are most likely to suffer from dehydration secondary to coughs?

   A. young children and clients with cardiac disease
   B. the elderly and clients with renal disease
   C. young children and the elderly
   D. young adults and clients with respiratory dysfunction

3. Which of the following expectorants is administered in drops and given in fluids?

   A. saturated solution of potassium iodide
   B. diphenhydramine
   C. codeine
   D. dextromethorphan HBr

4. One common complication of using narcotic cough suppressants is

   A. CNS excitation
   B. respiratory depression
   C. bronchial dilation
   D. constipation

5. The most widely used non-narcotic cough suppressant is

   A. ammonium chloride
   B. dextromethorphan HBr
   C. benzonatate
   D. guaifenesin

6. Which of the following medications should not be used in children due to the possibility that hypothyroidism may occur?
   A. potassium iodide
   B. diphenhydramine
   C. dextromethorphan
   D. guaifenesin

7. Guaifenesin is used as
   A. an expectorant to liquefy respiratory tract secretions
   B. a decongestant to dry respiratory tract secretions
   C. an antihistamine to dry respiratory tract secretions
   D. an antitussive agent to liquefy respiratory tract secretions

Critical Thinking Exercises

1. List major types of expectorants and antitussive agents, and describe their effects and contraindications.

   _____

   _____

   _____

   _____

   _____

2. Create a teaching plan for your client taking antitussive and expectorant medications, including interventions and ways to maintain client safety.

   _____

   _____

   _____

   _____

   _____

3. Review and provide information on how the physician determines whether to use an expectorant or an antitussive agent.

   _____

   _____

   _____

   _____

   _____

CHAPTER 16 Bronchodilators and Other Respiratory Agents

Objectives

After reading Chapter 16 of *Pharmacological Aspects of Nursing Care,* 7th edition, the student will be able to:

- State the mechanisms of action of adrenergic stimulants and xanthine derivatives.
- State how beclomethasone dipropionate works to prevent asthma attacks.
- Contrast and compare the administration routes, adverse effects, and expected therapeutic actions of bronchodilators, adrenergic stimulants, xanthine derivatives, and mucolytic agents.
- Discuss the interactions between bronchodilators and other medications.
- Discuss nursing interventions associated with the administration of bronchodilators and other respiratory agents.

Matching

Match the following terms with their correct definitions.

_____ 1. chronic obstructive pulmonary disease (COPD)

_____ 2. sensitized mast cells

_____ 3. xanthine derivatives

_____ 4. zafirlukast

_____ 5. beractant

_____ 6. status asthmaticus

_____ 7. colfosceril palmitate

_____ 8. acetylcysteine

A. these drugs produce diuresis

B. a synthetic lung surfactant administered directly into the trachea

C. the most commonly used mucolytic agent

D. these release histamine and leukotrienes

E. a collection of respiratory diseases that impairs respiratory function

F. the first leukotriene receptor antagonists used for the treatment of asthma

G. a natural surfactant derived from the lungs of cows

H. an unrelieved asthma attack, lasting for an extended period of time; may be fatal

True or False

Place T or F on the line before each statement.

_____ 1. Leukotrienes contribute to airway edema, smooth muscle constriction, and altered cellular activity.

_____ 2. Acetylcysteine reacts unfavorably with copper, rubber, and iron.

_____ 3. The therapeutic serum level of theophylline is 10–20 mcg/mL.

_____ 4. Aminophylline may be administered by intravenous push.

_____ 5. Clients on sympathomimetics can safely use monoamine oxidase inhibitors.

_____ 6. Analeptic medications are used to treat drug-induced respiratory depression.

Multiple Choice

Circle the best answer for each of the following questions. There is only one answer to each question.

1. Clients using albuterol inhalers should be cautioned to use only as directed because overdosing can cause

   A. bronchodilation and tachycardia

   B. bradycardia and tachypnea

   C. tachycardia and bronchoconstriction

   D. visual changes and palpitations

2. Anticholinergic drugs antagonize the action of acetylcholine, resulting in which of the following conditions?

   A. bronchodilation

   B. hypotension

   C. hypertension

   D. lethargy

3. Theophylline levels should be drawn at the peak of drug absorption. The optimal times for blood draws are

   A. 3 hours after immediate-release medication, 4 hours after sustained-release medication

   B. 1–2 hours after immediate-release medication, 4 hours after sustained-release medication

   C. 4 hours after immediate-release medication, 6 hours after sustained-release medication

   D. 2 hours after immediate-release medication, 6 hours after sustained-release medication

4. Clients receiving sympathomimetic agents may have potentiation of which of the following medications?

   A. tricyclic antidepressants

   B. monoamine oxidase inhibitors

   C. acetylcholinesterase

   D. prazosin

5. Clients receiving bronchodilators should have increased fluids, unless contraindicated. How much fluid should the client receive daily?

   A. 1200–1800 mL

   B. 3000–4000 mL

   C. 1800–2500 mL

   D. 2000–3000 mL

6. When caring for clients with chronic obstructive pulmonary disease, the nurse should take which of the following special precautions?

   A. administer high levels of oxygen for dyspnea episodes

   B. keep head of bed elevated to increase ease of breathing

   C. restrict fluids so client does not choke

   D. instruct client to install dehumidifier in his or her home

   E. instruct client to avoid pursed-lip breathing, as this tires client

7. Clients who have received epinephrine should have which of the following?

   A. increased fluids

   B. intubation

   C. the injection site should be massaged after intramuscular administration

   D. monitor to detect bradycardia

8. Clients receiving isoproterenol HCl or isoproterenol sulfate should be notified of which of the following?

   A. The medication may cause somnolence

   B. The medication may be safely used by clients with cardiac conditions

   C. Solutions may be administered

   D. Their sputum and/or saliva may turn pink when the drug is given by inhalation

Critical Thinking Exercises

1. List major types of bronchodilators and other respiratory agents, and describe their effects and contraindications.

   _____

   _____

   _____

   _____

   _____

2. Create a care plan for your client taking bronchodilators, adrenergic stimulants, xanthine derivatives, and mucolytic agents.

_____

_____

_____

_____

_____

3. Review and provide information on how respiratory diseases and conditions are diagnosed and classified.

_____

_____

_____

_____

_____

CHAPTER 17 *Cardiac Stimulants and Depressants*

Objectives

After reading Chapter 17 of *Pharmacological Aspects of Nursing Care,* 7th edition, the student will be able to:

- Identify the major types of cardiac stimulants, glycosides, calcium channel antagonists, and antiarrhythmic agents, along with the therapeutic actions and adverse effects of each medication.
- Discuss the interactions between cardiac glycosides and other medications.
- Discuss nursing interventions associated with the administration of cardiac medications.
- Distinguish between positive and negative inotropic effects, positive and negative chronotropic effects, and positive and negative dromotropic effects on heart agents.
- Describe the mechanisms of action involved in antiarrhythmic agents.
- Discuss the most common adverse effects related to the administration of cardiac stimulants and cardiac glycosides.

Matching

Match the following terms with their correct definitions.

_____ 1. cardiac glycoside

_____ 2. positive inotropic effect

_____ 3. negative inotropic effect

_____ 4. positive chronotropic effect

_____ 5. negative chronotropic effect

_____ 6. positive dromotropic effect

_____ 7. antiarrhythmic medication

_____ 8. sinoatrial (SA) node

_____ 9. atrioventricular (AV) node

_____ 10. automaticity

A. the pacemaker of the heart

B. increases the force of the heart's contractions

C. the ability of the heart to spontaneously initiate electrical activity

D. reduces the force of the heart's contractions

E. increases the heart rate by altering the rate of impulse formation at the sinoatrial (SA) node

F. Digoxin is an example of these drugs that decrease the velocity of electrical conduction and prolong the refractory period in the atrioventricular (AV) conduction system

G. an increase in the rate of electrical conduction

H. a decrease in the rate of electrical conduction

I. this structure generates the electrical impulse

J. these drugs work by decreasing automaticity, altering conduction rates, or altering the refractory period between cardiac contractions

True or False

Place T or F on the line before each statement.

_____ 1. Digoxin toxicity may occur in 20–30% of clients.

_____ 2. Potassium chloride is not administered for the treatment of digoxin toxicity.

_____ 3. Disopyramide may be safely used by clients with a history of myasthenia gravis.

_____ 4. Ventricular tachycardia, couplets, and premature ventricular contractions may be treated with mexiletine HCl.

_____ 5. Clients taking quinidine should use sunscreen due to increased photosensitivity.

Multiple Choice

Circle the best answer for each of the following questions. There is only one answer to each question.

1. Your client is experiencing premature ventricular contractions. You would expect which medication to be prescribed to treat this condition?

   A. acebutolol
   B. amiodarone HCl
   C. flecainide acetate
   D. dopamine HCl

2. Pulmonary toxicity is a potential adverse effect of which of the following agents?

   A. verapamil HCl
   B. diltiazem HCl
   C. calcium channel blocking agents
   D. amiodarone HCl

3. Bretylium commonly causes orthostatic hypotension, nausea, and vomiting. Which nursing intervention minimizes these effects?

   A. the administration of oxygen
   B. putting the client's bed in the Trendelenburg position
   C. the administration of antiemetics
   D. keeping the client in a supine position for 10–30 minutes

4. One complication of using cardiac glycosides is toxicity. Which of the following symptoms may be reported by the client?

   A. central nervous system (CNS) depression
   B. respiratory depression
   C. yellow or green-tinted vision
   D. constipation

5. Tissue necrosis from the infusion of dopamine or norepinephrine is treated with an infusion of

   A. phentolamine
   B. adenosine
   C. bretylium tosylate
   D. milrinone lactate

6. Which of the following medications is effective for cardioversion in terminating paraoxysmal supraventricular tachycardia (PSVT)?

   A. potassium iodide
   B. adenosine
   C. isradipine
   D. disopyramide

7. Your client's digoxin serum level is 3.5 ng/mL. Your first action should be to

   A. assess vital signs
   B. notify the health care provider
   C. raise the head of the client's bed
   D. administer oxygen

8. Oxytocic drugs, when used concurrently with adrenergic stimulants in obstetric clients to correct hypotension, may cause complications. What serious complication may occur?

   A. life-threatening arrhythmias
   B. peripheral vasoconstriction
   C. sympathomimetic response
   D. hypertension, resulting in cerebral blood vessel rupture postpartum

9. Dobutamine and dopamine HCl should not be mixed with which of these solutions?

   A. magnesium sulfate
   B. sodium chloride
   C. sodium bicarbonate
   D. hydrogen peroxide

10. Your client's pulse rate is 52 beats per minute, with a digoxin level of 2.5 ng/nl and a potassium level of 2.8 mEq/L. You would anticipate which of the following agents to be prescribed to treat this client?

    A. amrinone lactate
    B. quinidine
    C. digoxin
    D. digoxin immune fab

11. Before the administration of each dose of cardiac glycoside medication is given, the nurse should

    A. check the radial pulse for 30 seconds
    B. check the apical pulse for one full minute
    C. hold the medication if the client's heart rate is > 60 bpm
    D. check the client's serum digoxin level

12. The absorption of digoxin may be affected by
    A. bulk-forming laxatives
    B. stool softeners
    C. antihistamines
    D. corticosteroids

Critical Thinking Exercises

1. List major types of cardiac stimulants and depressants, and describe their effects and contraindications.

   _____

   _____

   _____

   _____

   _____

2. Create a care plan for your client taking cardiac glycoside, sympathomimetic agents, and antiarrhythmic agents, including interventions and ways to maintain client safety.

   _____

   _____

   _____

   _____

   _____

3. Describe how cardiac glycoside, sympathomimetic agents, and antiarrhythmic agents work to improve cardiac function.

   _____

   _____

   _____

   _____

CHAPTER 18 Agents That Dilate Blood Vessels

Objectives

After reading Chapter 18 of *Pharmacological Aspects of Nursing Care,* 7th edition, the student will be able to:

- Discuss the therapeutic actions and adverse effects of nitrates.
- Discuss the interactions between nitrates and other medications.
- Discuss nursing interventions associated with the administration of cardiac medications.
- Discuss the mechanisms of action involved in using coronary vasodilators.
- Discuss the most common adverse effects related to the administration of nitrates.
- Describe the procedure to be used for the administration of amyl nitrate and topical nitroglycerin products.

Matching

Match the following terms with their correct definitions.

_____ 1. nitrates

_____ 2. amyl nitrate

_____ 3. mibefradil dihydrochloride

_____ 4. nitroglycerin

A. decreases cardiac workload and increases cardiac blood supply

B. decreases peripheral vascular resistance and lowers blood pressure

C. a volatile liquid in a glass capsule that is crushed and directly inhaled

D. increases the blood flow and redistribution of blood to ischemic areas

True or False

Place T or F on the line before each statement.

_____ 1. Pure nitroglycerin is highly stable and does not require any special precautions.

_____ 2. Pentaerythritol tetranitrate is used prophylactically for the prevention of angina.

_____ 3. Nitrates may be safely used by clients with a history of glaucoma.

_____ 4. Acute myocardial infarction (MI) and angina may be treated with nitroglycerin.

_____ 5. Clients usually experience no major side effects from nitroglycerin administration.

_____ 6. Nitroglycerin may be administered through oral, transdermal, and intravenous routes.

Multiple Choice

Circle the best answer for each of the following questions. There is only one answer to each question.

1. The number one cause of death in the United States is
   - A. ischemic heart disease
   - B. stroke
   - C. breast cancer
   - D. lung cancer

2. Which of the following medications may cause a burning sensation in the mouth after administration?
   - A. amyl nitrate
   - B. isosorbide dinitrate
   - C. pentaerythritol tetranitrate
   - D. sublingual nitroglycerin

3. Nitroglycerin, given sublingually, usually relieves anginal chest pain within _____ minutes in 90% of clients.

   A. 10   C. 5
   B. 15   D. 2

4. One use of vasodilators is for the treatment of obstructive peripheral vascular disorders. Which of the following is an obstructive disorder?

   A. Raynaud's phenomenon   C. arteriosclerosis obliterans
   B. angina   D. atherosclerosis

5. Which of the following medications is used for the treatment of vasospastic disorders?

   A. mibefradil dihydrochloride   C. papaverine
   B. niacinamide   D. milrinone lactate

6. Which of the following medications is an effective treatment for intermittent claudication?

   A. nylidrin HCl   C. cilostazol
   B. cyclandelate   D. disopyramide

7. Which spasmolytic acts similarly in manner to papaverine?

   A. isoxsuprine HCl   C. niacinamide
   B. trandolapril HCl   D. cyclandelate

8. Intravenous nitroglycerin must be administered

   A. through central venous access   C. only to hemodynamically stable clients
   B. using an infusion pump   D. using reinforced plastic containers

9. Prinzmetal's angina is different in that
   A. anginal pain occurs when patient is at rest
   B. sublingual nitroglycerin does not work effectively
   C. it is a precursor to acute myocardial infarction
   D. anginal pain only occurs early in the morning

10. Your client is prescribed nitroglycerin topical disc. You should include which of the following instructions when teaching your client about this medication?
    A. remove previous disc after applying current dose
    B. rise slowly from a sitting or lying position
    C. apply before first meal of the day
    D. burning sensation in the mouth is a positive sign of potency

Critical Thinking Exercises

1. List the types of vasodilators, and describe their effects and contraindications.

   _____

   _____

   _____

   _____

   _____

2. Create a care plan for your client taking vasodilators, including interventions and ways to maintain client safety. Specify techniques for promoting safety of the feet and lower extremities.

_____

_____

_____

_____

_____

3. Describe how nitrate and non-nitrate medications work to improve peripheral blood flow.

_____

_____

_____

_____

_____

4. Describe major side effects of vasodilators and interventions to minimize these effects.

_____

_____

_____

_____

_____

CHAPTER 19 Agents Affecting Blood Clotting

Objectives

After reading Chapter 19 of *Pharmacological Aspects of Nursing Care,* 7th edition, the student will be able to:

- Discuss the therapeutic actions and adverse effects of medications that may induce bleeding or delay coagulation.
- Discuss the interactions between anticoagulants and other medications.
- Discuss nursing interventions associated with the administration of anticoagulants, thrombolytic enzymes, alteplase, anistreplase, and heparin.
- Describe the mechanisms of action involved in using anticoagulants, thrombolytic enzymes, alteplase, anistreplase, and heparin.
- Discuss the most common adverse effects related to the administration of heparin and other anticoagulants.
- Describe the procedure to be used for the administration of subcutaneous heparin.
- Discuss which laboratory results should be monitored for each particular type of medication that affects blood clotting.

Matching

Match the following terms with their correct definitions.

_____ 1. thrombus

_____ 2. hemostatic agents

_____ 3. pentoxifylline

_____ 4. tPA

_____ 5. aprotinin

A. used to stop the flow of blood in cases of excessive bleeding

B. tissue plasminogen activator created by recombinant DNA technology

C. a hemorrheologic agent used to increase the flexibility of red blood cells, which reduces aggregation

D. a blood clot

E. given intravenously and prophylactically to prevent blood loss in clients undergoing coronary artery bypass graft

True or False

Place T or F on the line before each statement.

_____ 1. Anticoagulants may exert a fibrinolytic effect on existing blood clots.

_____ 2. Enoxaparin is currently approved for intravenous use.

_____ 3. The evidence of oral anticoagulants appears almost immediately after administration.

_____ 4. Clients usually experience no major side effects from the administration of anticoagulants if they follow their health care providers' recommendations.

_____ 5. Warfarin may be administered through oral, transdermal, and intravenous routes.

Multiple Choice

Circle the best answer for each of the following questions. There is only one answer to each question.

1. Alteplase recombinant is used to treat acute ischemic cerebrovascular accidents. It is most effective in decreasing residual effects of a stroke if given
   A. 24 hours after the stroke
   B. within the first 3 hours following the stroke
   C. for 8 hours following the stroke
   D. instead of heparin to treat this type of stroke

2. Which of the following medications may cause increased oral anticoagulant activity?

   A. ethyl alcohol
   B. barbiturates
   C. hydantoins
   D. carbamazepine

3. Which of the following herbals/drugs will help the body metabolize anticoagulants more quickly?

   A. carbamazepine
   B. antacids
   C. oral contraceptives
   D. clarithromycin

4. One complication that may occur from the overuse of anticoagulants is

   A. excessive hypoprothrombinemia
   B. angina
   C. low platelet counts
   D. increased red blood cell count

5. Which of the following medications are used for the treatment of platelet aggregation?

   A. glycoprotein IIb/IIIa inhibitors
      and ticlopidine
   B. acetaminophen and ticlopidine
   C. papaverine and heparin
   D. warfarin and acetaminophen

6. Eptifibatide is a synthetic version of a protein found in rattlesnake venom. What condition(s) is it used to treat?

   A. bleeding disorders
   B. acute myocardial infarction
   C. stroke
   D. hypertension

7. Which antithrombolytic must not be administered intramuscularly due to the high risk of hematoma formation?

   A. warfarin
   B. heparin
   C. ketoprofen
   D. tenecteplase

8. Alteplase is commonly administered as an antithrombotic therapy for clients suffering acute stroke or myocardial infarction (MI). The maximum recommended dose is 150 mg. What serious complication may occur if the dose exceeds the maximum?

   A. acute MI
   B. increased intracranial pressure
   C. intracranial hemorrhage
   D. thromboembolus

9. Which of the following medications may be administered to clients with hemophilia after surgery or tooth extraction?

   A. pentoxifylline
   B. tranexamic acid
   C. thrombin
   D. streptokinase

10. What laboratory values should be monitored for clients receiving intravenous heparin therapy?

   A. prothrombin time (PT)
   B. international normalized ratio (INR)
   C. activated partial thromboplastin time (APTT)
   D. erythrocyte sedimentation rate

11. Clients receiving anticoagulant therapy should be instructed to

   A. monitor their capillary bleeding time
   B. wear a medical alert bracelet
   C. decrease their fluid intake
   D. take vitamin K if receiving heparin

Critical Thinking Exercises

1. Discuss the types of anticoagulants, and describe their effects and contraindications.

   _____

   _____

   _____

   _____

   _____

2. Create a care plan for your client taking anticoagulants and antithrombotics, including interventions and client education that should be performed. Specify techniques for promoting the safety of the client.

_____

_____

_____

_____

_____

3. Differentiate how anticoagulants and antithrombotic medications work to improve peripheral blood flow.

_____

_____

_____

_____

_____

4. Describe major side effects of anticoagulants and interventions to minimize these effects.

_____

_____

_____

_____

_____

CHAPTER 20 Diuretics and Antihypertensives

Objectives

After reading Chapter 20 of *Pharmacological Aspects of Nursing Care,* 7th edition, the student will be able to:

- Discuss the mechanisms of action and side effects of the major classes of diuretics.
- Discuss the mechanisms of action and side effects of the major classes of antihypertensives.
- Discuss the interactions between antihypertensives, diuretics, and other medications.
- Apply nursing interventions associated with the administration of antihypertensives and diuretics.
- Present nursing interventions to minimize adverse effects of long-term antihypertensive use.
- Describe sodium-restricted diets and goals of dietary modifications.

Matching

Match the following terms with their correct definitions.

_____ 1. loop diuretics

_____ 2. thiazide diuretics

_____ 3. metabolic alkalosis

_____ 4. methyldopate HCl

_____ 5. carbonic anhydrase

A. these medications prevent reabsorption at the loop of Henle

B. this enzyme is found in the kidneys and eyes, and promotes reabsorption of sodium and bicarbonate from the proximal tubule

C. this medication is metabolized to alpha-methylnorepinephrine

D. excessive chloride depletion may lead to this condition

E. these medications may cause hypokalemia

True or False

Place T or F on the line before each statement.

_____ 1. A hypertensive emergency exists when diastolic blood pressure is greater than 120 and there is evidence of renal, cardiac, or central nervous system (CNS) damage.

_____ 2. Respiratory depression and bradycardia may occur after the administration of beta adrenergic blockers.

_____ 3. One of the main reasons clients stop taking antihypertensive medications is the presence of side effects.

_____ 4. Minoxidil is usually given with a beta-blocker.

_____ 5. Antihypertensives and diuretics may be administered through oral, transdermal, and intravenous routes.

Multiple Choice

Circle the best answer for each of the following questions. There is only one answer to each question.

1. A normal adult client filters _____ of fluid daily.
   - A. 120 liters
   - B. 100 liters
   - C. 180 liters
   - D. 150 liters

2. Which of the following medications may cause the growth of fine body hair within 3–6 weeks of starting therapy?
   - A. nitroglycerin
   - B. betaxolol
   - C. benazepril HCl
   - D. minoxidil

3. Which of the following potassium-sparing diuretics may be used in combination with a thiazide if the client is receiving a cardiac glycoside?

   A. spironolactone
   B. hydrochlorothiazide
   C. furosemide
   D. atenolol

4. One complication of mecamylamine HCl use is

   A. ileus
   B. asthma
   C. low platelet counts
   D. hypertension

5. Which of the following medications is used for the treatment of severe hypertension as well as malignant hypertension?

   A. diazoxide
   B. amlodipine
   C. mecamylamine HCl
   D. hydralazine

6. This medication may cause venous pooling when the client is in an upright position.

   A. valsartan
   B. clonidine
   C. prazosin
   D. sodium nitroprusside

7. Which of the following conditions is characterized by significant hypotension and syncope with sudden loss of consciousness if prazosin, terazosin, or doxazosin are administered too rapidly?

   A. first-dose effect
   B. hypertensive crisis
   C. bronchospasm
   D. drug toxicity

8. One side effect of this medication is a dry cough.

   A. benazepril HCl
   B. captopril
   C. felodipine
   D. doxazosin mesylate

9. What is the most common symptom of hypertension?

   A. diarrhea
   B. insomnia
   C. constipation
   D. headache

10. What laboratory values should be monitored for clients receiving thiazide diuretics?

    A. sodium
    B. potassium
    C. magnesium
    D. bicarbonate

11. Thiazide diuretics may cause _____ in clients with diabetes or gout.

    A. hypoglycemia
    B. ecchymosis
    C. hyperglycemia
    D. hypouricemia

12. A condition characterized by excessive extracellular fluid, which may accumulate in the abdomen, is called

    A. ascites
    B. edema
    C. peripheral vasodilation
    D. hepatic edema

Critical Thinking Exercises

1. Present the types of diuretics, and describe their effects and contraindications.

_____

_____

_____

_____

_____

2. Create a care plan for your client taking diuretics and antihypertensives, including nursing interventions and client education that should be performed. Specify techniques for promoting client safety.

_____

_____

_____

_____

_____

3. Explain how antihypertensive medications work to improve peripheral blood flow.

_____

_____

_____

_____

_____

4. Describe how diuretics work to decrease blood pressure.

_____

_____

_____

_____

_____

CHAPTER 21 Agents Used in the Treatment of Hyperlipidemia

Objectives

After reading Chapter 21 of *Pharmacological Aspects of Nursing Care,* 7th edition, the student will be able to:

- Discuss the major classes, mechanisms of action, and side effects of agents used for hyperlipidemia.
- Describe the role diet plays in the prevention of atherosclerosis and hyperlipidemia.
- Discuss the interactions between antihyperlipidemic medications and other medications.
- Apply nursing interventions associated with the administration of antihyperlipidemic medications.
- Describe low-fat diets and the goals of dietary modifications.
- Discuss dietary sources of cholesterol.
- Describe saturated, unsaturated, monounsaturated, and polyunsaturated fats.

Matching

Match the following terms with their correct definitions.

_____ 1. atherosclerosis

_____ 2. high-density lipoproteins (HDL)

_____ 3. low-density lipoproteins (LDL)

_____ 4. very low-density lipoproteins (VLDL)

_____ 5. chylomicrons

A. these lipoproteins contain the highest proportion of lipids and are the least dense

B. secreted in the liver; triglycerides are partially derived from dietary sources

C. these contain the greatest proportion of cholesterol of all lipoproteins

D. excessive buildup of cholesterol and plaque on blood vessel walls

E. the smallest lipoprotein with the highest proportion of protein

True or False

Place T or F on the line before each statement.

_____ 1. Very low-density lipoprotein (VLDL) and low-density lipoprotein (LDL) levels are most important in the promotion of atherosclerosis.

_____ 2. The use of antihyperlipidemic medications significantly improves mortality rates.

_____ 3. Monounsaturated fats are the healthiest type of fat.

_____ 4. Cholestyramine is safe to administer with other medications.

_____ 5. Antihyperlipidemics may be administered through oral routes only.

Multiple Choice

Circle the best answer for each of the following questions. There is only one answer to each question.

1. An important adverse effect of simvastatin administration is

   A. hypolipidemia

   B. the lowering of low-density lipoprotein (LDL) levels

   C. hepatic functional changes

   D. the raising of high-density lipoprotein (HDL) levels

2. Which of the following medications increases, or does not change, triglyceride levels?

   A. cholestyramine resin
   B. fluvastatin

   C. nicotinic acid
   D. probucol

3. Which of the following medications must be used with extreme caution in clients with extensive histories of alcohol consumption or liver disease?

   A. dextrothyroxine sodium
   B. cholestyramine

   C. HMG-CoA reductase inhibitors
   D. colesevelam HCl

4. One complication of dextrothyroxine sodium is

   A. increased frequency and severity of anginal attacks
   B. hypernatremia

   C. hypotension
   D. hypertension

5. Which of the following medications is used as a binding agent of bile acids?

   A. cholestyramine
   B. nicotinic acid

   C. probucol
   D. fosinopril

6. Nicotinic acid administration may cause flushing and pruritus. Which of the following medications blocks prostaglandins and helps to relieve these symptoms?

   A. gemfibrozil
   B. acetaminophen

   C. acetylsalicylic acid
   D. sodium nitroprusside

7. Which of the following conditions should be reported immediately to the health care provider when using HMG-CoA reductase inhibitors?

   A. increased energy level
   B. constipation

   C. peripheral edema
   D. unexplained muscle pain

Critical Thinking Exercises

1. Discuss the types of agents used for hyperlipidemia, and describe their effects and contraindications.

   _____

   _____

   _____

   _____

   _____

2. Create a care and teaching plan for your client taking antihyperlipidemic agents, including nursing interventions and client education that should be performed. Specify techniques for promoting client safety.

   _____

   _____

   _____

   _____

   _____

3. Explain how the different antihyperlipidemic medications work to improve peripheral blood flow and decrease atherosclerosis.

_____

_____

_____

_____

_____

4. Make a diet plan for clients who are trying to lower their cholesterol.

_____

_____

_____

_____

_____

CHAPTER 22 Agents Used to Treat Anemias

Objectives

After reading Chapter 22 of *Pharmacological Aspects of Nursing Care,* 7th edition, the student will be able to:

- Describe the symptoms of anemia.
- Discuss the groups of individuals most at risk for anemia.
- Describe red blood cell shapes: normocytic, microcytic, hypochromic, and megaloblastic.
- Discuss the signs of iron toxicity and treatment options.
- Describe diets rich in iron and vitamin B_{12}, and the goals of dietary modifications.

Matching

Match the following terms with their correct definitions.

_____ 1. vitamin B_{12a}

_____ 2. anemia

_____ 3. the ferrous form of iron

_____ 4. vitamin B_{12}

_____ 5. erythropoietin

A. this agent stimulates red blood cell production

B. hydroxocobalamin

C. the most absorbable form of iron

D. decreases in red blood cells associated with a decrease in hemoglobin concentration

E. cyanocobalamin

True or False

Place T or F on the line before each statement.

_____ 1. The ferrous form of iron is absorbed three times more readily by the human body.

_____ 2. Intramuscular injections of iron dextran may cause sterile abscesses and hematomas.

_____ 3. The maximum amount of iron dextran that should be administered intramuscularly to one site is 3 mL.

_____ 4. The average diet provides 100 mcg of folic acid daily.

Multiple Choice

Circle the best answer for each of the following questions. There is only one answer to each question.

1. Tissue hypoxia caused by anemia may lead to

   A. muscle excitation
   B. hypokalemia
   C. angina pectoris
   D. drowsiness

2. Clients most likely to experience iron-deficiency anemia are

   A. toddlers
   B. preschoolers
   C. school-age children
   D. adolescents

3. The most common cause of iron-deficiency anemia is

   A. nutritional deficiency
   B. hematological disorders
   C. chemotherapy administration
   D. heredity

4. The major site of gastrointestinal absorption of iron is

   A. the sigmoid colon
   B. the proximal portion of the large intestine
   C. the proximal portion of the small intestine
   D. the distal portion of the stomach

5. Iron-deficient red blood cells are shaped

    A. macrocytic

    B. hypochromic and microcytic

    C. normocytic

    D. microcytic

6. Normally, 5–10% of ingested iron is absorbed by the body. This amount may increase to _____% in clients with serious iron-deficiency anemia.

    A. 30–50

    B. 15–20

    C. 10–15

    D. 20–30

7. When instructing clients who are at the greatest risk of developing iron-deficiency anemia about foods rich in iron, the nurse should include

    A. yellow vegetables

    B. citrus fruits

    C. dark green, leafy vegetables

    D. chicken breast meat

8. Clients with anemia caused by vitamin B_{12} deficiency may exhibit symptoms of

    A. diarrhea

    B. constipation

    C. bradycardia

    D. numbness and tingling of the extremities

9. Which of the following is a chelating agent used to remove excess iron from the body?

    A. deferoxamine mesylate

    B. hydroxocobalamin

    C. cyanocobalamin

    D. ferrous fumarate

10. What is one caution that the nurse should provide the client receiving deferoxamine mesylate?

    A. pernicious anemia may result from treatment

    B. their urine may be colored red from the medication

    C. their skin may turn orange

    D. they may develop angina

Critical Thinking Exercises

1. Discuss the types of anemia, and describe their signs, symptoms, and treatment.

_____

_____

_____

_____

_____

2. Using the Internet, research the most current statistics concerning the incidence of the different types of anemia. Identify specific groups of individuals with the greatest incidence.

_____

_____

_____

_____

_____

3. After researching question 2, discuss the characteristics of the groups targeted with anemia and explain why these groups have the greatest incidence.

_____

_____

_____

_____

_____

4. Create a teaching plan for your client taking iron supplements, including nursing interventions. Specify techniques for promoting client safety.

_____

_____

_____

_____

_____

5. Discuss the complications of chronic blood transfusions and how they are treated. Do these complications change life expectancy? Can these complications be prevented?

_____

_____

_____

_____

_____

CHAPTER 23 Vitamins, Minerals, and Other Nutritional Agents

Objectives

After reading Chapter 23 of *Pharmacological Aspects of Nursing Care*, 7th edition, the student will be able to:

- Discuss the major vitamins and minerals, their mechanisms of action, and the amounts needed for adequate health.
- Discuss the roles of protein, fat, and carbohydrates in nutrition.
- Discuss fat-soluble and water-soluble vitamins, and how deficiencies may occur.
- Demonstrate understanding of the causes of hypokalemia, hyperkalemia, and hypernatremia.
- Describe therapeutic diets and the goals of dietary modifications.

Matching

Match the following terms with their correct definitions.

_____ 1. vitamins

_____ 2. minerals

_____ 3. fat-soluble vitamins

_____ 4. water-soluble vitamins

_____ 5. lipoproteins

_____ 6. proteins

_____ 7. carbohydrates

_____ 8. fats

_____ 9. hypernatremia

A. thiamine, folic acid, and vitamin C are examples of these nutrients needed by the body

B. sugars and starches

C. concentrated source of fatty acids, 9 kcal/g

D. proteins and fat bound together to facilitate transport

E. serum sodium concentration is greater than 145 mEq/L

F. substances needed for chemical reactions, maintenance of health, and growth

G. this nutrient is 4 kcal/g and is used for the synthesis, maintenance, and repair of body tissues

H. divided into two groups: major elements and micro elements

I. vitamins A, D, E, and K; stored by the body

True or False

Place T or F on the line before each statement.

_____ 1. There are 50 nutrients required by the body, but only 10 are "leader" nutrients.

_____ 2. Proteins are composed of amino acids. Of 22 amino acids, only 8 are considered essential.

_____ 3. Hyponatremia appears first in the client as excessively dry skin.

_____ 4. Children should receive supplemental fluoride until age 10.

_____ 5. Copper, chromium, and selenium are examples of trace elements.

Multiple Choice

Circle the best answer for each of the following questions. There is only one answer to each question.

1. The predominant positively charged intracellular ion is
   A. potassium
   B. sodium
   C. plasma
   D. magnesium

2. The predominant positively charged extracellular ion is

   A. potassium   C. plasma
   B. sodium   D. magnesium

3. Excessive sodium loss from the body is most commonly caused by

   A. hypertension   C. severe diarrhea and vomiting
   B. peripheral edema   D. polyuria

4. Which of the following is a cause of hypokalemia?

   A. nausea   C. hypernatremia
   B. hyperaldosteronism   D. respiratory alkalosis

5. Hypokalemia may cause cardiac arrhythmias. Another serious complication that may occur is

   A. convulsions   C. sensitization to digitalis-like drugs, making cardiotoxicity more likely upon administration of those drugs

   B. muscle cramps   D. osteoporosis

6. Treatment for acute hyperkalemia is usually directed at reversing adverse cardiac events. Which of the following medications may be used to correct the hyperkalemia?

   A. calcium gluconate   C. sodium fluoride
   B. triameterene   D. sodium polystyrene sulfonate

7. Clients receiving calcium supplements may develop which of the following conditions?

   A. hypocalcemia   C. hyperuricemia
   B. hyperalbuminemia   D. hyperphosphatemia

8. Only about _____% of dietary iron is absorbed by the body.

   A. 30   C. 10
   B. 20   D. 5

9. Clients on renal dialysis may develop hypermagnesia. The treatment for hypermagnesia in renal clients is

   A. calcium supplements   C. sodium polystyrene sulfonate
   B. aluminum   D. sorbitol

10. Trace elements are important for many bodily functions. Which of the following is a trace element?

    A. sodium   C. chloride
    B. magnesium   D. copper

11. Treatment of potassium extravasation is directed at reducing vasospasm and diluting the concentration of potassium in the tissues. Which of the following medications may be effective?

    A. procaine penicillin   C. lidocaine
    B. hyaluronidase   D. sodium polystyrene sulfonate

12. Because of the high concentration of glucose in TPN, TPN should be infused through a central venous access device. The nurse understands that this places the client at high risk for

    A. hypoglycemia   C. deficient fluid volume
    B. infection   D. malnutrition

Critical Thinking Exercises

1. Research the types of vitamins and minerals, comparing the recommended daily intakes with common intake practices.

   _____

   _____

   _____

   _____

   _____

2. Describe the effects of vitamins, minerals, carbohydrates, proteins, and fats, along with their contraindications.

   _____

   _____

   _____

   _____

   _____

3. Create a nutritional and weight-loss plan for a client with renal failure and hypertension. Provide educational materials for your client.

   _____

   _____

   _____

   _____

   _____

CHAPTER 24 Agents Used to Treat Hyperacidity and Gastroesophageal Reflux Disease

Objectives

After reading Chapter 24 of *Pharmacological Aspects of Nursing Care,* 7th edition, the student will be able to:

■ Discuss the types, therapeutic actions, and adverse effects of medications used to treat gastrointestinal disorders.

■ Apply the nursing process to patient teaching (i.e., what would you teach the client about hyperchlorhydria?).

■ Discuss three prescription medications that should not be administered with antacids, and explain why.

■ Discuss the difference between systemic and nonsystemic antacid administration.

Matching

Match the following terms with their correct definitions.

_____ 1. hyperchlorhydria

_____ 2. parietal cells

_____ 3. peptic ulcer

_____ 4. antacids

_____ 5. antibiotics

A. antacids may decrease the effectiveness of these

B. the overproduction of hydrochloric acid

C. alkaline chemical agents used to provide relief from hyperacidity and peptic ulcer disease (PUD)

D. the erosion of the gastrointestinal lining; may be caused by H. pylori

E. secrete hydrochloric acid

True or False

Place T or F on the line before each statement.

_____ 1. Antacid activity may be decreased by administering antibiotics at the same time.

_____ 2. The most commonly used systemic drug used to treat hyperchlorhydria is simethicone.

_____ 3. Simethicone should not be used during an acute attack of gastric distress.

_____ 4. Sodium bicarbonate may be safely used in all patients experiencing gastric distress.

Multiple Choice

Circle the best answer for each of the following questions. There is only one answer to each question.

1. Antacids are used to
   A. heal gastric ulcers
   B. heal erosions of the esophagus
   C. treat the pain associated with peptic ulcer disease (PUD)
   D. control the heartburn associated with gastroesophageal reflux disease (GERD)

2. Clients taking magnesium oxide or magnesium hydroxide should be monitored for
   A. diarrhea
   B. leukopenia
   C. hypertension
   D. hypocalcemia

3. The client receiving antacids should not have antibiotics administered within _____ hour(s) of antibiotics.

   A. one
   B. six

   C. three
   D. four

4. Which of the following medications should be avoided if the client has an ulcer?

   A. acetaminophen
   B. antacids

   C. aspirin
   D. proton-pump inhibitors

5. Which of the following medications is ulcerogenic and should be avoided?

   A. acetaminophen
   B. allopurinol

   C. cyclobenzaprine
   D. indomethacin

Critical Thinking Exercises

1. Describe the effects of systemic and nonsystemic antacids.

   _____

   _____

   _____

   _____

   _____

2. Create a care plan for a client with peptic ulcer disease, including interventions and how you would evaluate your goals.

   _____

   _____

   _____

   _____

   _____

CHAPTER 25 Emetics and Antiemetics

Objectives

After reading Chapter 25 of *Pharmacological Aspects of Nursing Care,* 7th edition, the student will be able to:

■ Discuss the types, therapeutic actions, and adverse effects of emetic and antiemetic medications.

■ Discuss histamine H_2 antagonists and their uses.

■ Apply nursing interventions associated with the administration of emetics and antiemetics.

Matching

Match the following terms with their correct definitions.

_____ 1. emetics

_____ 2. antiemetics

_____ 3. histamine H_2-receptor antagonists

_____ 4. proton-pump inhibitors

_____ 5. promethazine

_____ 6. ondansetron

A. given to prevent and treat nausea and vomiting

B. a 5-HT3 antagonist used to treat nausea and vomiting associated with chemotherapy

C. given to produce vomiting

D. inhibit the action of histamine in parietal cells

E. block the enzyme system at the secretory surface of the parietal cells in the stomach in order to block the secretion of hydrochloric acid

F. phenothiazine antiemetic

True or False

Place T or F on the line before each statement.

_____ 1. Common antiemetics include scopolamine, metoclopramide (Reglan), loperamide (Imodium), and difenoxin and atropine (Motofen).

_____ 2. Cimetidine may cause gynecomastia and impotence.

_____ 3. Extrapyramidal reactions frequently occur when administering pancreatic enzymes.

_____ 4. Histamine H_2 blockers are safe to give to clients of any age.

_____ 5. Increased pharmacological effects may occur when some medications are administered concurrently with cimetidine.

_____ 6. Proton-pump inhibitors are used for the treatment of gastroesophageal reflux disease (GERD).

Multiple Choice

Circle the best answer for each of the following questions. There is only one answer to each question.

1. The most common adverse effect associated with ondansetron is

   A. nausea
   B. diarrhea
   C. somnolence
   D. hypotension

2. Which of the following medications is used to treat gastroesophageal reflux disease (GERD)?

   A. esomeprazole
   B. granisetron HCl
   C. fexofenadine
   D. promethazine

3. Ondansetron is administered primarily for which of the following conditions?
   A. GERD
   B. constipation
   C. peptic ulcer disease
   D. chemotherapy-induced nausea

4. Nausea may be caused by all of the following *except*?
   A. hormonal changes
   B. intense pain
   C. relaxation
   D. stress

5. Anticholinergic agents are contraindicated in clients with which of the following?
   A. bradydysrhythmias
   B. acute renal failure
   C. peptic ulcer disease
   D. increased intraocular pressure

6. Chemotherapy-induced nausea and vomiting is most commonly treated with
   A. neuroleptics
   B. prokinetic agents
   C. serotonin-blocking agents
   D. antihistamines

7. Antihistamines may cause which of the following adverse effects?
   A. increased risk of urinary retention in client with benign prostatic hypertrophy
   B. increased urinary frequency resulting from overactive bladder
   C. worsening of diarrhea in client with Crohn's disease
   D. increased perspiration associated with elevated glucose levels

8. Chlorpromazine and droperidol (Inapsine) may cause serious adverse effects. Which of the following may occur?
   A. hypertension
   B. QT prolongation
   C. decreased plasma cholesterol
   D. nausea and vomiting

9. This medication is used to stimulate acetylcholine in order to increase gastric emptying.
   A. metoclopramide
   B. droperidol
   C. ondansetron
   D. aprepitant

10. Promethazine HCl, when given intravenously, is incompatible with which of the following solutions?
    A. lactated ringers
    B. dextrose
    C. 0.9% normal saline
    D. Ringer's solution

Critical Thinking Exercises

1. Research and list the classes of emetics and antiemetics. Prepare a presentation in which you discuss their mechanisms of action and provide two examples of each.

_____

_____

_____

_____

_____

2. Research and describe the approval history of the major types of antihistamines and anticholinergic medications used as antiemetics.

_____

_____

_____

_____

_____

3. Create a care plan for your client taking antiemetics, including interventions and ways to maintain hydration.

_____

_____

_____

_____

_____

CHAPTER 26 Laxatives and Antidiarrheals

Objectives

After reading Chapter 26 of *Pharmacological Aspects of Nursing Care,* 7th edition, the student will be able to:

■ Discuss the differences between stimulant, lubricant, and bulk-forming laxatives.

■ Define laxatives and antidiarrheal agents.

■ Discuss the major types of laxatives used for constipation, their therapeutic actions, and the adverse effects of each medication.

■ Discuss the interactions between laxatives and other medications.

■ Discuss antidiarrheal agents, their therapeutic actions, and the adverse effects of each medication.

■ Apply nursing interventions associated with the administration of laxatives and antidiarrheal agents.

Matching

Match the following terms with their correct definitions.

_____ 1. stool softeners

_____ 2. bulk-forming laxatives

_____ 3. constipation

_____ 4. suppositories

_____ 5. lubricant laxatives

_____ 6. diarrhea

_____ 7. antidiarrheals

A. condition in which the passage of feces is slow or nonexistent

B. facilitate the passage of fecal mass through the intestine by maintaining hydration of the fecal mass

C. stimulant agents that promote elimination

D. absorb fluid and swell in the intestine, promoting peristalsis

E. permit easier mixing of fat and fluids in the fecal mass

F. this class of medication reduces gastrointestinal motility

G. abnormally frequent passage of watery stools

True or False

Place T or F on the line before each statement.

_____ 1. The central nervous system (CNS) may be affected by the administration of antidiarrheals.

_____ 2. Clients experiencing acute abdominal pain should take a laxative prior to notifying their physician.

_____ 3. Clients may become addicted to suppository use.

_____ 4. Laxatives are drugs intended to facilitate the passage of food from the stomach through the intestines to be eliminated.

_____ 5. Adsorbents such as bismuth may prevent the absorption of other oral medications.

Multiple Choice

Circle the best answer for each of the following questions. There is only one answer to each question.

1. Bulk-forming laxatives should always be administered with
   A. increased volumes of fluid
   B. eight ounces of water
   C. eight ounces of juice
   D. decreased volumes of fluid

2. Clients taking antidiarrheal medications containing opiates should be monitored for

   A. dependence
   B. respiratory depression
   C. no special monitoring is needed
   D. seizures

3. Polyethylene glycol is a solution used to induce a diarrheal state to promote cleansing of the bowel. The mechanism of action of polyethylene glycol is

   A. it lubricates and promotes water retention in the fecal mass
   B. it possesses adsorbent properties
   C. it causes a large volume of water to be retained in the colon
   D. it provides bulk-forming agents to help form stool

4. Causes of diarrhea may include

   A. physical activity
   B. medications
   C. decreased fluid intake
   D. psychosis

5. Clients should use caution when driving or operating heavy equipment when taking which of the following medications?

   A. loperamide hydrochloride
   B. diphenoxylate hydrochloride with atropine sulfate
   C. psyllium hydrophilic mucilloid
   D. docusate sodium

6. Which of the following laxatives may discolor the stool?

   A. psyllium hydrophilic mucilloid
   B. psyllium
   C. phenolphthalein
   D. misoprostol

7. After the administration of saline laxatives, geriatric clients may experience adverse effects such as

   A. central nervous system (CNS) excitation
   B. central nervous system (CNS) depression
   C. renal insufficiency
   D. severe headache

Critical Thinking Exercises

1. Discuss major types of bulk-forming, lubricant, and saline laxatives, as well as stool softeners. Include their mechanisms of action, and provide two examples of each.

   _____

   _____

   _____

   _____

2. Create a teaching plan for your client taking laxatives and antidiarrheal agents.

   _____

   _____

   _____

   _____

   _____

3. Create a visual presentation of the special needs of older clients and children taking laxatives and antidiarrheals.

_____

_____

_____

_____

_____

CHAPTER 27 Central Nervous System Sedatives and Hypnotics

Objectives

After reading Chapter 27 of *Pharmacological Aspects of Nursing Care,* 7th edition, the student will be able to:

- Discuss the types, therapeutic actions, and adverse effects of barbiturates, sedatives, and hypnotic medications.
- Discuss the differences between barbiturates, sedatives, and hypnotic agents.
- Describe the expected therapeutic effects of barbiturates, sedatives, and hypnotic agents.
- Discuss nursing interventions associated with the administration of barbiturates, sedatives, and hypnotic agents.

Matching

Match the following terms with their correct definitions.

_____ 1. sedatives

_____ 2. benzodiazepines

_____ 3. barbiturates

_____ 4. hypnotics

A. these medications cause relaxation and promote sleep

B. central nervous system depressant that potentiates gamma-aminobutyric acid (GABA) mediated neural inhibition

C. reduce nervousness and anxiety without causing sleep; also called anxiolytics

D. this type of medication produces central nervous system depression and anticonvulsant activity

True or False

Place T or F on the line before each statement.

_____ 1. There are over 2,500 barbiturates approved for use in the United States.

_____ 2. Respiratory and vasomotor centers may be depressed by high doses of barbiturates.

_____ 3. Exfoliative dermatitis may occur with the administration of benzodiazepines.

_____ 4. Sedatives are safe to give to most clients.

_____ 5. Chloral hydrate causes depressed rapid eye movement (REM) sleep and produces medication "hangovers."

_____ 6. Most nonprescription sleep aids have an antihistamine in their formulation.

_____ 7. Alcohol (ethanol) is a stimulant.

_____ 8. Barbiturates and benzodiazepines are non-habit-forming.

_____ 9. Anterograde amnesia and paradoxical reactions may be induced by the administration of pentobarbital.

_____ 10. Clients with prolonged use of barbiturates may increase vitamin D requirements.

Multiple Choice

Circle the best answer for each of the following questions. There is only one answer to each question.

1. Which of the following medications is a nonbarbiturate, nonbenzodiazepine hypnotic?
   - A. zolpidem tartrate
   - B. lorazepam
   - C. chloral hydrate
   - D. midazolam

2. Clients receiving benzodiazepines as sleep aids should be monitored for which of the following adverse effects?

   A. insomnia
   B. gastric upset
   C. dependency
   D. respiratory depression

3. Benzodiazepines are commonly used for the treatment of

   A. insomnia
   B. hysteria
   C. anxiety
   D. psychosis

4. This medication may not be safely used by clients taking drugs metabolized by microsomal enzymes, such as warfarin.

   A. flurazepam
   B. temazepam
   C. triazolam
   D. phenobarbital

5. Your client is receiving eszopiclone, and you understand that this medication is indicated for

   A. pre-procedural sedation
   B. longer-term treatment for sleep disorders
   C. adjunct treatment for epilepsy
   D. treatment of anxiety disorders

6. Common signs of barbiturate toxicity include

   A. deep sleep, coma
   B. hypotension, excitation
   C. pupil constriction, cyanosis
   D. A, B, and C
   E. A and C

7. Which of the following sedative medications is non-habit-forming?

   A. temazepam
   B. diazepam
   C. trazodone
   D. zaleplon

8. Your postoperative client on the nursing unit of the local hospital is receiving triazolam. Your actions with this client would include all of the following *except*

   A. raising the side rails on the bed
   B. lowering the bed to the lowest position
   C. administering opioid analgesic for incision pain
   D. having the client sign advanced directives

9. Rapid discontinuation of these mediations may cause coma, convulsions, or death.

   A. barbiturates
   B. benzodiazepines
   C. anxiolytics
   D. sleep aids

10. After the administration of barbiturates, the nurse should monitor clients for

   A. renal insufficiency
   B. hypersensitivity reactions, especially in clients with asthma
   C. hepatic dysfunction
   D. nausea and vomiting

Critical Thinking Exercises

1. List major types of barbiturates, sedatives, and hypnotic medications. Discuss their mechanisms of action, and provide two examples of each.

   _____

   _____

   _____

   _____

   _____

2. List major types of benzodiazepines, and describe their effects and contraindications.

_____

_____

_____

_____

_____

3. Create a care plan for your client taking sedatives and hypnotics, including interventions and ways to maintain client safety.

_____

_____

_____

_____

_____

4. Research information clients may utilize to determine the signs, symptoms, and effects of medications used to treat anxiety and convulsant disorders.

_____

_____

_____

_____

_____

CHAPTER 28 Anxiolytics and Other Agents Used to Treat Psychiatric Conditions

Objectives

After reading Chapter 28 of *Pharmacological Aspects of Nursing Care,* 7th edition, the student will be able to:

■ Discuss the major types, therapeutic actions, and adverse effects of psychotropic medications.

■ Discuss the differences between barbiturates, antihistamines, and antipsychotic agents.

■ Describe the expected therapeutic effects of barbiturates, antihistamines, and antipsychotic agents.

■ Discuss nursing interventions associated with the administration of barbiturates, antihistamines, and antipsychotic agents.

Matching

Match the following terms with their correct definitions.

_____ 1. psychotropic drugs

_____ 2. anxiety, psychoses, and affective disorders

_____ 3. neuroleptics

_____ 4. affective disorders

_____ 5. tardive dyskinesia

_____ 6. norepinephrine

_____ 7. barbiturates

_____ 8. serotonin

A. suppress spontaneous movement and complex behaviors

B. changes in mood

C. used to treat emotional and mental disorders

D. this medication is used primarily for the treatment of insomnia

E. psychotropic drugs are used to treat these conditions

F. neurotransmitter thought to be responsible for depressive states

G. extrapyramidal symptoms that do not appear until the client has been taking antipsychotic agents for over two years

H. neurotransmitter responsible for mood

Multiple Choice

Circle the best answer for each of the following questions. There is only one answer to each question.

1. Clozapine is effective for the treatment of mental illness and lacks many adverse effects. One serious complication that may occur with the use of clozapine is

   A. thrombocytopenia
   B. agranulocytosis
   C. leukopenia
   D. neutropenia

2. Clients taking antipsychotic agents may develop fever, muscle rigidity, altered consciousness, and altered vital signs. What is the name of this condition?

   A. autonomic dysreflexia
   B. extrapyramidal symptoms
   C. neuroleptic malignant syndrome
   D. malignant hypertension

3. Affective disorders are characterized by

   A. depression
   B. changes in behavior
   C. changes in mood
   D. increased libido

4. An excess of norepinephrine may cause

   A. anxiety   C. depression

   B. psychosis   D. mania

5. This tricyclic drug is used to treat obsessive-compulsive disorder.

   A. clomipramine HCl   C. imipramine

   B. amitriptyline   D. fluoxetine

6. The biogenic hypothesis suggests that

   A. depression results from serotonin and catecholamine deficiencies

   B. alterations in neurotransmitters in the central nervous system (CNS) are responsible for depression

   C. affective disorders are primarily psychosomatic

   D. psychotropic medications will be discontinued after 90 days

7. What do almost all antidepressants have in common?

   A. they have a long half-life   C. they are for short-term use

   B. they begin having a therapeutic effect in one week   D. all are safe for use among elderly clients

Critical Thinking Exercises

1. Form a study group to discuss nursing assessments and interventions for clients receiving anxiolytics. Discuss their mechanisms of action, and provide two examples of each.

   _____

   _____

   _____

   _____

   _____

2. Create a care plan for your client taking monoamine oxidase inhibitors, including interventions and ways to maintain client safety.

   _____

   _____

   _____

   _____

   _____

3. Research and provide information on how mental disorders are classified and diagnosed.

_____

_____

_____

_____

_____

CHAPTER 29 Central Nervous System Stimulants Used to Treat Attention-Deficit Hyperactivity Disorder and Agents Used to Treat Alzheimer's Disease

Objectives

After reading Chapter 29 of *Pharmacological Aspects of Nursing Care,* 7th edition, the student will be able to:

- Identify the types, therapeutic actions, and adverse effects of anorectic and non-anorectic agent medications.
- Discuss the differences between anorectic agents and stimulants.
- Describe the expected therapeutic effects of anorectics, analeptics, and stimulants.
- Discuss nursing interventions associated with the administration of anorectics, analeptics, and stimulants.

Matching

Match the following terms with their correct definitions.

_____ 1. tacrine HCl

_____ 2. amphetamines

_____ 3. atomoxetine HCl

_____ 4. analeptics

_____ 5. anorectic agents

_____ 6. ergoloid mesylate

_____ 7. doxapram HCl

_____ 8. narcolepsy

A. used for the treatment of respiratory depression caused by narcotics or other central nervous system depressants

B. used to improve cognitive skills and motivation in clients over the age of 60

C. inhibit cholinesterase, thereby increasing acetylcholine

D. may be used in the treatment of attention-deficit/attention-deficit hyperactivity disorder (ADD/ADHD) and narcolepsy

E. a condition characterized by attacks of sleep occurring throughout the day

F. classified as controlled substances, these medications are both short- and long-acting

G. used for the treatment of ADHD to improve attention span

H. arterial blood gases must be monitored prior to initiating therapy with this medication

True or False

Place T or F on the line before each statement.

_____ 1. Methylphenidate HCl is safe to administer concurrently with monoamine oxidase inhibitors.

_____ 2. Arterial blood gases should be closely monitored prior to initiating therapy with citrated caffeine.

_____ 3. Clients taking pemoline should have frequent hepatic monitoring.

_____ 4. Laryngospasms may occur with the administration of anorectic medications.

_____ 5. One cup of brewed coffee has 120 mg of caffeine.

_____ 6. Non-anorectic medications may be safely administered in patients with hypertension or cardiac disease if closely monitored.

Multiple Choice

Circle the best answer for each of the following questions. There is only one answer to each question.

1. This non-anorectic central nervous system stimulant may result in psychological dependence, multiple drug interactions, blood disorders, and increased seizures.

   A. diethylpropion HCl
   B. doxapram HCl
   C. methylphenidate HCl
   D. methamphetamine HCl

2. Atomoxetine HCl is contraindicated in clients receiving

   A. monoamine oxidase inhibitors
   B. other controlled substances
   C. treatment for fibrocystic breast disease
   D. supraventricular tachycardia

3. Your client is receiving pemoline and, as a result, should be monitored for

   A. bradycardia
   B. central nervous system (CNS) stimulation
   C. liver toxicity
   D. narcolepsy

4. Clients who take amphetamines for long periods of time must be gradually weaned off of the medication to prevent which of the following conditions?

   A. lethargy
   B. depression
   C. convulsions
   D. fatigue

5. Your client is diagnosed with mild Alzheimer's disease. The health care provider discusses the use of a cholinesterase inhibitor to treat the client. This would include

   A. rivastigmine
   B. donepezil
   C. galantamine
   D. methylphenidate HCl

6. Memantine is used to treat Alzheimer's disease by its action of

   A. altering levels of acetylcholine
   B. inhibiting cholinesterase
   C. inhibiting acetylcholinesterase
   D. blocking dopamine

7. Clients receiving medication for the treatment of Alzheimer's disease should be instructed to

   A. take on an empty stomach for full effects
   B. avoid vitamin supplements
   C. follow up with health care provider every six months
   D. take with food to help decrease adverse gastric effects

Critical Thinking Exercises

1. Research and explain how different mental disorders are classified and diagnosed.

   _____

   _____

   _____

   _____

   _____

2. Create a care plan for your client taking analeptics and anorectics, including interventions and ways to maintain client safety.

_____

_____

_____

_____

_____

3. Research information clients may utilize to determine the signs, symptoms, and effects of medications used to treat attention-deficit disorders.

_____

_____

_____

_____

_____

CHAPTER 30 Agents Used in Musculoskeletal Disorders

Objectives

After reading Chapter 30 of *Pharmacological Aspects of Nursing Care,* 7th edition, the student will be able to:

- Identify the types, therapeutic actions, and adverse effects of neuromuscular blocking medications.
- Discuss the differences between neuromuscular blocking agents and skeletal muscle relaxants.
- Differentiate agents that may potentiate the effects of neuromuscular agents.
- Identify nursing interventions associated with the administration of neuromuscular blocking agents and skeletal muscle relaxants.

Matching

Match the following terms with their correct definitions.

_____ 1. neuromuscular junction

_____ 2. streptomycin

_____ 3. neostigmine

_____ 4. acetylcholine

_____ 5. neuromuscular blockade

_____ 6. cholinesterase

_____ 7. neurotransmitter

_____ 8. spondylitis

A. the space between motor nerves and each muscle cell

B. intentional paralysis of a client using medications to paralyze the skeletal muscles

C. neurotransmitter needed to initiate muscle contraction

D. this medication is an antidotal drug to neuromuscular blocking agents

E. enzyme needed to break down acetylcholine

F. this medication may potentiate some neuromuscular blocking agents

G. fusion of joints in an abnormal position

H. chemical messenger

True or False

Place T or F on the line before each statement.

_____ 1. Phenytoin may increase the effects of neuromuscular blocking agents.

_____ 2. Tubocurarine chloride may be mixed with barbiturates in a syringe prior to administration.

_____ 3. Clients with myasthenia gravis may be experiencing an autoimmune response, according to recent evidence.

_____ 4. Valium may precipitate if given by the intravenous drip method.

_____ 5. Baclofen is used primarily for clients experiencing spasms related to muscular dystrophy.

_____ 6. Central nervous system medications may be safely administered concurrently with skeletal muscle relaxants.

Multiple Choice

Circle the best answer for each of the following questions. There is only one answer to each question.

1. The preferred administration method of centrally acting skeletal muscle relaxants is

   A. oral

   B. intradermal

   C. parenteral

   D. buccal

2. Adverse effects of skeletal muscle relaxants include

   A. nervousness and dizziness
   B. dizziness and tachycardia
   C. somnolence and bradycardia
   D. excitation and drowsiness

3. Which of the following medications is five times as strong as tubocurarine chloride?

   A. mivacurium chloride
   B. pancuronium bromide
   C. cyclobenzaprine HCl
   D. succinylcholine chloride

4. Clients who take certain centrally acting skeletal relaxants for long periods of time must be gradually weaned off of the medication. Which of the following conditions is baclofen used for?

   A. multiple sclerosis and spinal cord injuries
   B. depression and spinal tumors
   C. back pain and muscle atonia
   D. muscle fatigue and muscle spasms

5. This medication may increase the effects of neuromuscular blocking agents.

   A. antiarrhythmic agents
   B. antianginal medications
   C. analgesics
   D. methylphenidate HCl

6. Which of the following medications may cause hepatotoxicity?

   A. centrally acting skeletal muscle relaxants
   B. neuromuscular blocking agents
   C. direct-acting skeletal muscle relaxants
   D. paralytic agents

7. Adverse effects of anticholinesterase medications include

   A. salivation
   B. dry eyes
   C. tachycardia
   D. constipation

8. Ptosis means

   A. excessive drooling
   B. bloody sputum
   C. drooping eyelids
   D. crossed eyes

Critical Thinking Exercises

1. Research and explain how different musculoskeletal agents are used.

   _____

   _____

   _____

   _____

   _____

2. List major types of neuromuscular and skeletal muscle relaxant medications, and describe their effects and contraindications.

   _____

   _____

   _____

   _____

   _____

3. Create a care plan for your client taking centrally acting muscle relaxants, including interventions and ways to maintain client safety.

_____

_____

_____

_____

_____

CHAPTER 31 Anti-Parkinson Agents

Objectives

After reading Chapter 31 of *Pharmacological Aspects of Nursing Care,* 7th edition, the student will be able to:

- Identify the types, therapeutic actions, and adverse effects of medications used to treat Parkinson's disease.
- Discuss the differences between anticholinergic and dopaminergic agents.
- Describe the expected therapeutic effects of anticholinergic and dopaminergic agents.
- Identify nursing interventions and processes associated with the administration of major anti-Parkinson agents.

Matching

Match the following terms with their correct definitions.

_____ 1. amantadine HCl

_____ 2. antihistamines

_____ 3. carbidopa

_____ 4. belladonna derivatives

_____ 5. pyridoxine

_____ 6. bromocriptine mesylate

A. the first anticholinergic medication used

B. inhibits the dopa decarboxylase (DDC) enzyme

C. originally developed for treating viral disorders

D. may be used in clients who have developed a tolerance to levodopa

E. may be used for their sedating effect, without causing mental disturbances

F. facilitates the breakdown of levodopa to dopamine in peripheral circulation

True or False

Place T or F on the line before each statement.

_____ 1. Clients taking entacapone may also take monoamine oxidase inhibitors.

_____ 2. Psychological changes may occur with the administration of bromocriptine mesylate.

_____ 3. Clients taking tolcapone should have frequent hepatic monitoring.

_____ 4. Constipation may occur with the administration of cholinergic medications.

_____ 5. Cholinergic medications may cause difficulties in clients with glaucoma and prostatic hypertrophy.

_____ 6. Selegiline HCl may cause hypertension in clients.

_____ 7. Drug-induced Parkinsonism is usually caused by antihistamine administration.

_____ 8. Clients receiving medications for Parkinson's disease should consume a diet high in vitamin B_6.

Multiple Choice

Circle the best answer for each of the following questions. There is only one answer to each question.

1. This medication is commonly used for reducing the incidence and severity of drug-induced side effects of anti-Parkinson drugs.
   - A. amantadine HCl
   - B. entacapone
   - C. carbidopa-levodopa
   - D. methamphetamine HCl

2. Adverse effects of tolcapone include

   A. dysuria
   B. orthostatic hypotension

   C. hypertension
   D. bradycardia

3. Identify the medication that warrants increased monitoring of liver functions.

   A. selegiline HCl
   B. pergolide mesylate

   C. levodopa
   D. tolcapone

4. Clients who take anticholinergic medications for long periods of time may develop a tolerance to them. All of the following medications may be prescribed in the event that tolerance has developed *except*

   A. pergolide mesylate
   B. bromocriptine mesylate

   C. selegiline HCl
   D. diphenhydramine

5. Benztropine, given as a single daily dose, is best administered during this time of day.

   A. early morning
   B. midday

   C. bedtime
   D. noon

6. Which of the following medications is most effective for treating Parkinson's disease?

   A. levodopa
   B. selegiline

   C. amantadine
   D. pergolide mesylate

7. Parkinson's disease is characterized by

   A. atonia, paresthesia
   B. rigidity, muscle tremors, bradycardia

   C. lack of coordination, muscle tremors, rigidity
   D. all of the above

8. Anticholinergic medications should be used with caution in clients with
   A. cardiac disease and cataracts
   B. narrow-angle glaucoma and benign prostatic hypertrophy
   C. epilepsy and wide-angle glaucoma
   D. respiratory dysfunction and pyelonephritis

Critical Thinking Exercises

1. Describe major types of Parkinson's disease medications, and discuss their effects and contraindications.

   _____

   _____

   _____

   _____

   _____

2. Create a care plan for your client taking dopaminergic and anticholinergic medications, including interventions and ways to maintain client safety.

   _____

   _____

   _____

   _____

   _____

3. Research information about diet modifications that may be needed for clients with Parkinson's disease.

_____

_____

_____

_____

_____

CHAPTER 32 *Anticonvulsants*

Objectives

After reading Chapter 32 of *Pharmacological Aspects of Nursing Care,* 7th edition, the student will be able to:

- Describe the common signs and symptoms of seizure disorders.
- List the common manifestations of partial, generalized, and focal seizures.
- Provide the definition of epilepsy.
- Identify the major types, therapeutic actions, and adverse effects of anticonvulsant medications.
- Discuss the interactions between anticonvulsants and other medications.
- Identify nursing interventions associated with the administration of anticonvulsant agents.

Matching

Match the following terms with their correct definitions.

_____ 1. felbamate

_____ 2. acetazolamide

_____ 3. carbamazepine

_____ 4. absence seizure

_____ 5. generalized tonic-clonic seizure

_____ 6. diazepam

_____ 7. intractable seizures

_____ 8. psychomotor or temporal lobe seizures

A. this medication may increase the seizure threshold in clients with Lennox-Gastaut syndrome

B. potentiates the action of anticonvulsants used to treat absence and nonlocalized seizures

C. the usual drug of choice for treating status epilepticus

D. this medication is used primarily for the treatment of trigeminal neuralgia

E. seizures that do not respond to conventional pharmacological anticonvulsant therapy

F. petit mal seizure

G. grand mal seizure

H. usually begins as a blank stare followed by random activity

True or False

Place T or F on the line before each statement.

_____ 1. Phenytoin may be given by IV push at 100 mg/minute.

_____ 2. Carbamazepine levels should be monitored yearly in new clients.

_____ 3. Valproic acid may be administered to clients who are pregnant or planning to become pregnant.

_____ 4. Bone mass increases with long-term administration of phenytoin.

_____ 5. Valproic acid may be discontinued without any special precautions.

_____ 6. Valproic acid may alter thyroid function and urine ketone tests.

_____ 7. Drowsiness, ataxia, and unsteady gait usually decrease with continued use of clonazepam.

_____ 8. Ibuprofen may be safely administered concurrently with phenytoin.

Multiple Choice

Circle the best answer for each of the following questions. There is only one answer to each question.

1. Seizures may be characterized by all of the following *except*

    A. loss of consciousness
    B. psychological changes
    C. abnormal motor functions
    D. continence

2. Epilepsy is defined as

    A. many types of recurrent seizures characterized by excessive electrical discharge of nerves in the cerebral cortex
    B. a series of continuous seizures
    C. a cognitive impairment resulting from abnormal electrical activity
    D. a series of electrical impulses stimulating more than one area of the brain at a time

3. A focal lesion means that

    A. the client focuses on the seizure
    B. the client loses consciousness
    C. uncontrolled electrical discharges occur in a localized area of the central nervous system
    D. the seizures begin in a specific area

4. One complication of phenytoin therapy is

    A. leukocytopenia
    B. gingival hyperplasia
    C. anemia
    D. elevated erythrocyte sedimentation rate

5. Phenytoin may be safely administered intravenously with which of the following solutions?

    A. dextrose 5% in water (D5W)
    B. 0.9% normal sterile saline (NSS)
    C. lactated Ringer's
    D. 0.45% NSS

6. Fatal aplastic anemia may result from administration of which of the following medications?

    A. valproic acid
    B. fosphenytoin
    C. phenytoin
    D. carbamazepine

7. Carbamazepine reacts with _____ and may result in carbamazepine toxicity.

    A. erythromycin
    B. streptomycin
    C. penicillin
    D. fluoxetine

8. Synergistic effects may occur when administering two or more medications concurrently. Which of the following produce enhanced therapeutic effects?

    A. phenytoin and phenobarbital
    B. isoniazid and heparin
    C. clonazepam and valium
    D. disulfiram and warfarin

9. Clients with seizure disorders may experience

    A. auras
    B. urinary continence
    C. dyspepsia
    D. diarrhea

10. Safety precautions for clients with epilepsy include all of the following *except*

    A. suction apparatus
    B. placing the bed in the lowest position
    C. padded side rails
    D. diazepam at the bedside

Critical Thinking Exercises

1. List the major types of anticonvulsants, and describe their effects and contraindications.

   _____

   _____

   _____

   _____

   _____

2. Create a care plan for your client taking anticonvulsant medications, including interventions and ways to maintain client safety.

   _____

   _____

   _____

   _____

   _____

3. Identify nursing assessments and interventions for clients with epilepsy.

   _____

   _____

   _____

   _____

   _____

4. Research and provide information on how seizure disorders are classified and diagnosed.

   _____

   _____

   _____

   _____

   _____

CHAPTER 33 Substance Abuse

Objectives

After reading Chapter 33 of *Pharmacological Aspects of Nursing Care,* 7th edition, the student will be able to:

- Discuss the underlying causes of addiction.
- Explain the major characteristics of substance abuse, dependence, and tolerance.
- Discuss the major substances involved: alcohol, marijuana, central nervous system (CNS) stimulants, sedatives, opioids, hallucinogens, and nicotine.
- Compare and contrast the different medications used to treat substance abuse, along with their mechanisms of action, therapeutic effects, and adverse side effects.

Matching

Match the following terms with their correct definitions.

_____ 1. addiction	A. central nervous system (CNS) adapts to repeated substance use and suffers withdrawal symptoms if the substance is not used
_____ 2. psychological dependence	B. once tolerance develops to a certain substance, the tolerance extends to chemically related drugs
_____ 3. tolerance	C. biological condition where the body adapts to a substance and its repeated administration
_____ 4. physical dependence	D. overwhelming compulsion to participate in unhealthy behavior despite negative consequences
_____ 5. cross-tolerance	E. intense cravings (but not physical discomfort) cause a person to use a substance

True or False

Place T or F on the line before each statement.

_____ 1. All hallucinogens or psychedelic drugs are Schedule V drugs.

_____ 2. Withdrawal syndrome from cocaine is more intense than from alcohol abuse.

_____ 3. Clients who smoke and take oral contraceptives are five times more likely to suffer a fatal heart attack than nonsmokers.

_____ 4. Metabolites of delta-9-tetrahydrocannabinol (THC) may remain in the client's body for months or years.

_____ 5. Cocaine is a Schedule III drug.

Multiple Choice

Circle the best answer for each of the following questions. There is only one answer to each question.

1. The two most commonly abused drugs are
   A. alcohol and nicotine
   B. alcohol and marijuana
   C. nicotine and narcotics
   D. narcotics and alcohol

2. Clients who have developed physical dependence and are attempting to discontinue use of opioids may be prescribed which of the following medications to decrease withdrawal symptoms?

   A. oxazepam
   B. trazodone

   C. methadone
   D. lorazepam

3. Intravenous drug users are at high risk for contracting

   A. severe streptococcal infections
   B. hepatitis B

   C. staphylococcal infections
   D. herpes simplex type I

4. Chronic alcohol use may cause_____in clients.

   A. cirrhosis
   B. renal failure

   C. nausea
   D. edema

5. This medication inhibits acetaldehyde dehydrogenase and causes severe adverse effects if used improperly.

   A. mescaline
   B. methylphenidate

   C. disulfiram
   D. diphenhydramine HCl

6. According to current research trends, cigarette/nicotine use in adolescents has _____over the past 3 years.

   A. dramatically increased
   B. increased slightly

   C. remained the same
   D. steadily declined

7. With short-term use, high doses of _____ make the user feel euphoric, alert, and that he or she can do anything.

   A. barbiturates
   B. amphetamines

   C. hypnotics
   D. cannabinoids

8. This drug may produce flashbacks months or years after use.

   A. methylphenidate
   B. cocaine

   C. methamphetamine
   D. lysergic acid diethylamide (LSD)

9. The liver metabolizes alcohol at a rate of _____ per hour.

   A. 10 mL
   B. 15 mL

   C. 100 mL
   D. 50 mL

10. The effects of caffeine classify it as a _____.

    A. sedative
    B. central nervous system (CNS) stimulant

    C. diuretic
    D. hallucinogenic

11. Opioid withdrawal may present all of the following manifestations *except*

    A. violent yawning
    B. piloerection

    C. agitation
    D. mental depression

Critical Thinking Exercises

1. Research the agents identified in this chapter that may cause physical or psychological dependence or addiction, along with the current treatments for chemical dependence on these agents.

   _____

   _____

   _____

   _____

   _____

2. Visit a drug rehabilitation facility and discuss with a licensed counselor the effects of barbiturates, amphetamines, depressants, opioids, and hallucinogens that brought clients to the facility.

_____

_____

_____

_____

_____

3. Create a care plan for your client suffering withdrawal symptoms, including educational materials.

_____

_____

_____

_____

_____

CHAPTER 34 Autonomic Nervous System

Objectives

After reading Chapter 34 of *Pharmacological Aspects of Nursing Care,* 7th edition, the student will be able to:

- Discuss the differences between the autonomic and sympathetic nervous systems.
- Describe the locations and functions of alpha- and beta-adrenergic receptors.
- Discuss the types, therapeutic actions, and adverse effects of medications used as antispasmodics.
- Apply the nursing process to client teaching (i.e., what would you teach the client about antispasmodics and anticholinergics?).
- Discuss nursing interventions associated with the administration of antispasmodics.

Matching

Match the following terms with their correct definitions.

_____ 1. neurotransmitters

_____ 2. parasympathetic

_____ 3. somatic nervous system

_____ 4. sympathetic

_____ 5. ganglion

_____ 6. alpha$_1$ receptors

_____ 7. alpha$_2$ receptors

_____ 8. sympatholytics

_____ 9. beta$_1$-adrenergic receptors

_____ 10. beta$_2$-adrenergic receptors

A. the cholinergic branch of the autonomic nervous system (ANS)

B. a single-neuron system

C. the adrenergic branch of the autonomic nervous system

D. chemical messengers that transmit impulses

E. cluster of nerve cell bodies

F. these block or inhibit the responses of adrenergic neurotransmitters

G. located primarily in bronchial smooth muscles and in blood vessels in the heart, brain, and skeletal muscle

H. located on the presynaptic neuron

I. located primarily in the smooth muscle of peripheral blood vessels, urinary, and gastrointestinal (GI) sphincters

J. found in the smooth muscle of the heart and in fatty tissue

True or False

Place T or F on the line before each statement.

_____ 1. Cholinergic drugs mimic the actions of the parasympathetic nervous system (PNS).

_____ 2. The autonomic nervous system (ANS) has two divisions: the parasympathetic and sympathetic branches.

_____ 3. Sympathomimetics utilize catecholamines to transmit messages.

_____ 4. A positive inotropic effect is decreased heart rate.

_____ 5. No special considerations are needed when administering antispasmodics and anticholinergics to the elderly.

_____ 6. Antispasmodics work synergistically with acetylcholine to reduce gastrointestinal (GI) motility.

_____ 7. Belladonna alkaloids are able to cross the blood-brain barrier.

_____ 8. The "fight or flight" action is part of the sympathetic nervous system (SNS).

_____ 9. Norepinephrine and acetylcholine are neurotransmitters used in the ANS.

_____ 10. Clients should be cautioned about driving or operating heavy machinery while taking anticholinergics.

Multiple Choice

Circle the best answer for each of the following questions. There is only one answer to each question.

1. Common adverse effects of anticholinergic administration are

   A. dry mouth
   B. ototoxicity
   C. increased urinary output
   D. diaphoresis

2. Clients taking pyridostigmine should be monitored for

   A. lacrimation
   B. blurred vision
   C. accommodation spasms
   D. cholinergic crisis
   E. none of the above

3. Anticholinergic agents are used for all of the following *except*

   A. to relax smooth muscle in the bronchi
   B. eye surgery (preoperatively)
   C. to treat Parkinson's disease
   D. glaucoma

4. The client diagnosed with myasthenia gravis may be prescribed cholinergics to alter the structure of his or her nerve cells. Common medications include

   A. terbutaline
   B. metoprolol
   C. edrophonium
   D. epinephrine

5. The anticholinergic action of scopolamine may cause

   A. increased urinary output
   B. increased tear production
   C. bradycardia
   D. decreased pressure in the eye

6. A complication related to the administration of anticholinergics in high doses is

   A. tachycardia
   B. bradycardia
   C. diaphoresis
   D. decreased tolerance to temperature changes

7. Which of the following medications should be avoided if the client has narrow-angle glaucoma, renal disease, or prostatic hypertrophy?

   A. belladonna
   B. antacids
   C. cholinergics
   D. pyridostigmine

8. Propranolol, metoprolol, and atenolol are examples of what classification of drugs?

   A. cholinergic agents
   B. anticholinergic agents
   C. sympathomimetic agents
   D. beta-adrenergic blocking agents

9. Belladonna overdose is treated with the administration of _____ to reverse the anticholinergic effects.

   A. neostigmine methylsulfate
   B. physostigmine
   C. hyoscyamine sulfate
   D. atropine sulfate

10. Geriatric clients make up a large proportion of clients with Alzheimer's disease, glaucoma, and myasthenia gravis being treated with cholinergic agents. A common adverse effect in older adults taking this classification of medications is

    A. constipation
    B. diarrhea
    C. fluid retention
    D. hallucinations

Critical Thinking Exercises

1. Discuss major types of cholinergics, anticholinergics, antispasmodics, and sympathomimetic medications, along with their uses and mechanisms of action. Provide two examples of each.

_____

_____

_____

_____

_____

2. Describe the effects of cholinergics, anticholinergics, antispasmodics, and sympathomimetic medications.

_____

_____

_____

_____

_____

3. Create a care plan for your client taking antispasmodics, including interventions and how you would evaluate your goals.

_____

_____

_____

_____

_____

4. Research and describe interventions clients may utilize for the side effects of anticholinergic and sympathiomimetic medications.

_____

_____

_____

_____

_____

CHAPTER 35 Agents Affecting Thyroid, Parathyroid, and Pituitary Function

Objectives

After reading Chapter 35 of *Pharmacological Aspects of Nursing Care,* 7th edition, the student will be able to:

- Discuss the major classes, mechanisms of action, and side effects of agents used for thyroid and parathyroid disease.
- Discuss the role diet plays in the treatment of thyroid disease.
- Discuss the interactions between thyroid medications and other medications.
- Apply nursing interventions associated with the administration of antithyroid and parathyroid medications.
- Describe hypoparathyroidism, hyperparathyroidism, and pituitary diseases.
- Apply nursing interventions to clients receiving thyroid replacement medications.
- Describe which laboratory values should be monitored for particular diseases.

Matching

Match the following terms with their correct definitions.

_____ 1. levothyroxine sodium

_____ 2. desmopressin acetate

_____ 3. calcitonin

_____ 4. adrenocorticotropic hormone (ACTH)

_____ 5. liothyronine sodium

_____ 6. parathyroid hormone

_____ 7. diabetes insipidus

_____ 8. somatropin

A. a purely synthetic thyroid hormone

B. this hormone regulates serum calcium levels

C. hypopituitarism is treated with this medication

D. the most widely prescribed thyroid hormonal agent

E. reduces serum calcium by inhibiting bone resorption

F. a condition caused by a deficiency or absence of vasopressin

G. medication used to treat diabetes insipidus

H. corticotropin

True or False

Place T or F on the line before each statement.

_____ 1. Clients with diabetes insipidus have the same symptoms as clients with diabetes mellitus.

_____ 2. Clients with hypoparathyroidism may suffer from fatigue, paresthesias, and muscle pain upon contraction.

_____ 3. Clients receiving thyroid replacement medications should expect normal blood levels immediately after starting their medication.

_____ 4. Clients with hypothyroidism may be more sensitive to narcotics and barbiturates.

_____ 5. Diabetes insipidus may cause hypernatremia.

Multiple Choice

Circle the best answer for each of the following questions. There is only one answer to each question.

1. The synthesis of thyroid hormone is controlled by the

   A. hypothalamus

   B. anterior pituitary

   C. posterior pituitary

   D. thyroid

2. The release of thyroid stimulating hormone (TSH) is controlled by

    A. negative feedback
    B. positive feedback
    C. the autonomic nervous system (ANS)
    D. the central nervous system (CNS)

3. Which of the following medications is effective in controlling hyperthyroidism?

    A. propylthiouracil
    B. levothyroxine
    C. levothroid
    D. Synthroid

4. Liothyronine sodium and levothyroxine sodium are used to treat which of the following conditions?

    A. pituitary tumors
    B. hyperthyroidism
    C. hypothyroidism
    D. hypertension

5. Treatment for the acute phase of hypoparathyroidism consists of the administration of which of the following medications?

    A. sodium chloride
    B. potassium chloride
    C. calcium gluconate
    D. magnesium citrate

6. The synthetic form of vasopressin may be used for enuresis and the treatment of clients with hemophiliac disease. What mechanism of action occurs in hemophiliac clients?

    A. an increase in Factor III
    B. an increase in Factor X
    C. an increase in Factor VIII
    D. an increase in Factor VII

7. The administration of corticotropin may cause which of the following side effects?

    A. decreased red blood cell production
    B. diuresis
    C. hypersecretion of parathyroid hormone
    D. increased blood glucose in diabetic clients

8. Hyperpituitarism may result in which of the following conditions?

    A. dwarfism
    B. hypernatremia
    C. short stature
    D. giantism

9. What condition may occur if the client has vasopressin levels that are too high?

    A. polyuria
    B. constipation
    C. diuresis
    D. water intoxication

10. Which medication is an effective treatment for Paget's disease?

    A. etidronate disodium
    B. somatropin
    C. adrenocorticotropic hormone (ACTH)
    D. desmopressin acetate

Critical Thinking Exercises

1. Develop a teaching visual for the types of agents used to treat thyroid disease, and describe their effects and contraindications.

    _____

    _____

    _____

    _____

    _____

2. Create a care and teaching plan for your client taking thyroid agents, including nursing interventions and client education that should be performed. Specify techniques for promoting client safety.

_____

_____

_____

_____

_____

3. Present the specific thyroid hormones and explain their functions.

_____

_____

_____

_____

_____

4. Describe a thyroid storm and the necessary emergency treatment.

_____

_____

_____

_____

_____

CHAPTER 36 Agents Used to Treat Hyperglycemia and Hypoglycemia

Objectives

After reading Chapter 36 of *Pharmacological Aspects of Nursing Care,* 7th edition, the student will be able to:

- Describe the symptoms of hyperglycemia.
- Describe the symptoms of hypoglycemia.
- Discuss the groups of individuals most at risk for hyperglycemia.
- Discuss optimal blood glucose levels, according to the American Diabetes Association.
- Describe the function of insulin.
- Discuss short-, intermediate-, and long-acting insulin, along with their mechanisms of action.
- Demonstrate the procedure for administering and drawing up insulin.
- Describe diabetic diets and the goals of dietary modifications.

Matching

Match the following terms with their correct definitions.

_____ 1. neutral protamine Hagedorn (NPH) insulin

_____ 2. Type I diabetes (IDDM)

_____ 3. lipolysis

_____ 4. Type II diabetes (NIDDM)

_____ 5. regular insulin

_____ 6. retinopathy

_____ 8. long-acting insulin

_____ 9. insulin

A. secreted by alpha cells of the islets of Langerhans

B. onset of action in 60–150 minutes; lasts 4–12 hours

C. non-insulin dependent; usually adult onset

D. rapid-acting insulin; onset in 15–60 minutes

E. onset in 4–8 hours; lasts 14–24 hours

F. the breakdown of fats to fatty acids

H. a condition that may occur from uncontrolled blood glucose levels

I. secreted by the beta cells of the islets of Langerhans

True or False

Place T or F on the line before each statement.

_____ 1. Most oral hypoglycemic agents are sulfonylureas.

_____ 2. Meglitinides decrease blood sugar by stimulating insulin release from the working beta cells in the pancreas.

_____ 3. The most suitable oral hypoglycemic agent for clients with kidney dysfunction is rosiglitazone maleate.

_____ 4. Oral hypoglycemic agents are usually given first thing in the morning, before breakfast.

_____ 5. Lipodystrophy may occur if an infrequently used site is injected with insulin.

Multiple Choice

Circle the best answer for each of the following questions. There is only one answer to each question.

1. This oral hypoglycemic agent may exert a uricosuric effect.

   A. tolazamide
   B. glipizide
   C. acetohexamide
   D. glimepiride

2. This medication is a thiazide derivative used to treat hypoglycemia in clients with pancreatic cancer.

   A. diazoxide
   B. metformin HCl
   C. pioglitazone
   D. miglitol

3. The most significant adverse effect of glitazone administration is

   A. hypoglycemia
   B. diarrhea
   C. liver damage
   D. renal failure

4. These oral hypoglycemic agents slow the rise of blood glucose levels by slowing the breakdown of sugars and starches.

   A. regular insulin
   B. glitazones
   C. insulin
   D. chlorpropamide

5. This medication has the lowest incidence of adverse effects and the shortest duration of action.

   A. tolbutamide
   B. glipizide
   C. metformin HCl
   D. sulfonylurea

6. When drawing up insulin that needs to be mixed for administration, in which order is the insulin drawn up?

   A. long-acting, then short-acting insulin
   B. regular, then lente insulin
   C. ultralente, then intermediate-acting insulin
   D. order doesn't matter

7. Insulin should be injected with the needle at an angle of _____ degrees.

   A. 50
   B. 45
   C. 75
   D. 90

8. After mixing regular and neutral protamine Hagedorn (NPH) insulin, the insulin must be administered within _____ minutes.

   A. 60
   B. 20
   C. 15
   D. 30

9. If a known diabetic client is discovered unconscious, the standard of care is to treat him or her initially for

   A. hyperglycemia
   B. diabetic ketoacidosis
   C. hypoglycemia
   D. hypernatremia

10. When teaching a client about the administration of insulin, which of the following comments made by the client would indicate that more teaching is needed?

    A. "I have to insert the same amount of air into the insulin vial as the amount of insulin I need to withdraw."

    B. "I don't understand why I can't take my insulin in a pill like my grandfather does."

    C. "When using my abdomen for my insulin injection, I need to leave at least 1–2 inches from my belly button free from injections."

    D. "I should monitor my blood sugar before meals and before I go to bed at night."

Critical Thinking Exercises

1. Research the signs and symptoms of hyperglycemia, and why they occur.

   _____

   _____

   _____

   _____

   _____

2. Create a teaching plan for your client taking oral hypoglycemic agents, including nursing interventions. Specify techniques for promoting client safety.

   _____

   _____

   _____

   _____

   _____

3. Review and explain how hyperglycemia occurs, as well as how the body reacts to insulin and oral agents.

   _____

   _____

   _____

   _____

   _____

CHAPTER 37 Sex Hormones

Objectives

After reading Chapter 37 of *Pharmacological Aspects of Nursing Care*, 7th edition, the student will be able to:

- Describe the classes of sex hormones and provide an example of each.
- Discuss common estrogen and progesterone medications, and their uses.
- Describe the mechanisms of action of reproductive hormones and any side effects that may occur.
- Discuss oral contraceptives and their mechanisms of action.
- Apply teaching strategies to clients with difficulty conceiving.

Matching

Match the following terms with their correct definitions.

_____ 1. estrogen conjugated, oral

_____ 2. estrogen

_____ 3. human chorionic gonadotropin

_____ 4. testosterone

_____ 5. progesterone

_____ 6. luteinizing hormone

_____ 7. androgens

A. during pregnancy, this hormone is essential for maintenance of the placenta and embryo

B. the secretion of this hormone stimulates the development of the corpus luteum

C. conjugated estrogen made from pregnant mare urine

D. male sex hormones

E. substances capable of producing estrus and development of secondary sex characteristics

F. this hormone initiates spermatogenesis

G. secreted by the placenta

True or False

Place T or F on the line before each statement.

_____ 1. Testosterone is most effective when given orally.

_____ 2. Clients receiving testosterone may experience sodium and chloride retention.

_____ 3. Enovid is used to treat endometriosis.

_____ 4. Danacrine suppresses the output of gonadotropins from the pituitary gland.

_____ 5. Clients receiving ovulation stimulants have a 50% chance of having multiple births.

Multiple Choice

Circle the best answer for each of the following questions. There is only one answer to each question.

1. The use of estrogens has been shown to increase the risk of
   A. pregnancy
   B. stroke
   C. thromboembolism
   D. hormonal dysfunction

2. Which of the following medications may reduce the effectiveness of estrogens?
   A. carbamazepine
   B. corticosteroids
   C. insulin
   D. anticoagulants

3. Clients receiving estrogen therapy may need increased dosages of which of the following medications?

   A. nevirapine   C. oral hypoglycemics

   B. penicillin   D. hydantoin

4. The consistent inability to obtain and maintain an erection sufficient for sexual intercourse is called

   A. libido   C. psychosomatic

   B. erectile dysfunction   D. potency

5. Sildenafil citrate is the first medication for erectile dysfunction. What makes this medication different from other drugs used for impotence?

   A. the relaxation of smooth muscle in the penis is maintained for longer periods of time

   B. the results may be permanent

   C. it may be taken more than once per day

   D. it only works in response to sexual stimulation

6. Androgens may be used to treat

   A. hypergonadism   C. infertility in women

   B. inoperable prostate cancer   D. inoperable breast cancer

7. This medication is implanted as subcutaneous pellets.

   A. nandrolone phenpropionate   C. oxymetholone

   B. testosterone aqueous suspension   D. methyltestosterone

8. This medication is used primarily for treatment of benign prostatic hypertrophy.

   A. finasteride   C. oxymetholone

   B. nafarelin acetate   D. danacrine

9. This medication is a purified preparation of gonadotropins extracted from the urine of postmenopausal women.

   A. menotropin   C. levofloxacin

   B. clomiphene citrate   D. sildenafil citrate

Critical Thinking Exercises

1. Discuss the role of sex hormones in the development and maturation of the human body.

2. Create a teaching plan for your client taking oral contraceptive agents, including nursing interventions. Specify techniques for promoting client safety.

3. Prepare a handout that will educate nonmedical clients on how each medication works and what to expect from each particular therapy.

_____

_____

_____

_____

_____

CHAPTER 38 Agents Used in Obstetrical Care

Objectives

After reading Chapter 38 of *Pharmacological Aspects of Nursing Care,* 7th edition, the student will be able to:

- Discuss the groups of medications commonly used for obstetrical care, as well as the therapeutic actions and side effects of each.
- Discuss the desired actions, effects, and modes of administration for each medication commonly used in labor and delivery.
- Describe the function of oxytocin.
- Apply the nursing interventions to be employed for obstetrical clients.

Matching

Match the following terms with their correct definitions.

_____ 1. carboprost tromethamine

_____ 2. oxytocin

_____ 3. prostaglandin gel

A. secreted by the posterior pituitary, this increases the frequency and force of uterine contractions

B. this medication is used to prepare the cervix for delivery

C. this medication is used to initiate abortion

True or False

Place T or F on the line before each statement.

_____ 1. Hirsutism may occur when a client receives lactation suppressants.

_____ 2. Oxytocin initiates production of breast milk.

_____ 3. Tobacco, alcohol, and caffeine may be present in breast milk.

_____ 4. Most medications are safe for pregnant or lactating women.

Multiple Choice

Circle the best answer for each of the following questions. There is only one answer to each question.

1. The administration of this medication requires an infusion pump and careful observation of the client.
   A. dinoprostone
   B. ergonovine maleate
   C. oxytocin
   D. ritodrine HCl

2. The drug used to induce labor is
   A. terbutaline
   B. ritodrine HCl
   C. dinoprostone
   D. oxytocin

3. Ergonovine maleate is used intravenously to do which of the following?
   A. relax the uterus
   B. contract the uterus and stop postpartum bleeding
   C. prolong the gestational period
   D. induce labor

4. This medication is commonly used to inhibit preterm labor.
   A. terbutaline sulfate
   B. oxytocin
   C. Rh0(D) immune globulin
   D. methylergonovine maleate

5. This medication is a gel used to ripen the cervix of a woman having an induced labor.
   A. terbutaline sulfate
   B. methylergonovine maleate
   C. ritodrine HCl
   D. dinoprostone

Critical Thinking Exercises

1. Create a visual presentation of the common signs of labor, including interventions to assist the laboring woman.

   _____

   _____

   _____

   _____

   _____

2. Create a care plan for your client taking prostaglandins, oxytocin, and other obstetrical agents. Include nursing interventions and specify techniques for promoting client safety.

   _____

   _____

   _____

   _____

   _____

3. Research breast-feeding information and support groups.

   _____

   _____

   _____

   _____

4. Prepare a report on abortions, and reflect on the nurse's role before, during, and after an abortion.

   _____

   _____

   _____

   _____

CHAPTER 39 Agents That Affect Immunity

Objectives

After reading Chapter 39 of *Pharmacological Aspects of Nursing Care,* 7th edition, the student will be able to:

■ Describe the drugs most often used to stimulate the immune system, as well as their mechanisms of action, therapeutic effects, and side effects. Give an example of each.

■ Describe the drugs most often used to depress the immune system, as well as their mechanisms of action, therapeutic effects, and major side effects. Give an example of each.

■ Discuss the recommended childhood immunizations.

Matching

Match the following terms with their correct definitions.

_____ 1. vaccine

_____ 2. chicken pox

_____ 3. pneumonia

_____ 4. epinephrine

A. agent to be used for anaphylactic reactions from immunizations

B. the pneumococcal vaccine protects against this

C. the varicella vaccine is used to prevent this illness

D. a medication containing weakened or dead antigens

Multiple Choice

Circle the best answer for each of the following questions. There is only one answer to each question.

1. This medication may only be given intramuscularly.
   A. Rh$_0$(D) immune globulin
   B. hepatitis B immune globulin
   C. immune globulin
   D. gamma globulin

2. Immunocompromised and dialysis clients should have what special considerations when receiving influenza vaccines?
   A. they should not receive the vaccine if they are sensitive to chicken eggs
   B. they should not receive the vaccine if they are allergic to thimerosal
   C. they should receive double the normal adult dose
   D. they should receive the vaccine twice a year

3. One of the most effective immunosuppressant agents is
   A. ketoprofen
   B. mycophenolate mofetil
   C. epoetin alfa recombinant
   D. cyclosporine

4. A post-renal transplant client receives cyclosporine. Which of the following symptoms would indicate to the nurse that the cyclosporine was ineffective with this client?
   A. chills, tachycardia, tachypnea
   B. leukocytosis, fever, hypotension
   C. dysuria, leukopenia, ascites
   D. oliguria, edema, fever

5. This medication may cause potassium imbalances.
   A. tacrolimus
   B. basiliximab
   C. mycophenolate mofetil
   D. cyclosporine

6. Cyclosporine is commonly used to prevent rejection of transplanted organs but has several serious side effects. Which of the following is a side effect of this medication?
   A. nephrotoxicity
   B. decreased transaminase
   C. hypotension
   D. decreased reflexes

7. These agents are used as immunosuppressants in small doses.

    A. glucocorticoids   C. interferon

    B. antiviral agents   D. antineoplastics

8. The initial dose of cytomegalovirus immune globulin must be given within _____ hours of organ transplantation.

    A. 24   C. 48

    B. 36   D. 72

Critical Thinking Exercises

1. Design a teaching poster of the required precautions for clients who have undergone a bone marrow transplant.

2. Create a care plan for your client undergoing organ transplantation. Specify techniques for promoting pain relief and client safety.

3. Research the history of childhood immunizations to present as a report to the class.

CHAPTER 40 Agents Used in the Treatment of Cancer

Objectives

After reading Chapter 40 of *Pharmacological Aspects of Nursing Care,* 7th edition, the student will be able to:

- List the major classes of antineoplastics and give an example of an agent in each class
- Describe the therapeutic actions and adverse side effects of each class of antineoplastic agents.
- Discuss agents that may be used to control side effects of antineoplastic administration.

Matching

Match the following terms with their correct definitions.

_____ 1. chemotherapy

_____ 2. antineoplastic agents

_____ 3. alkylating agents

_____ 4. "rescue drugs"

_____ 5. methotrexate

_____ 6. biologic-response modifiers

A. the type of medication that may interfere with cell cycles

B. interferes with folic acid metabolism and causes increased uric acid levels

C. drugs used in combination with chemotherapy and adjuvant agents

D. the use of drug therapy to destroy malignant cells

E. this medication activates the client's own immune system

F. interferes with chemical structures of DNA and causes abnormal bonding

True or False

Place T or F on the line before each statement.

_____ 1. Epoetin is a synthetic version of erythropoietin that stimulates bone marrow to produce red blood cells.

_____ 2. Cisplatin may be given intravenously through infusion devices without any special precautions.

_____ 3. The client receiving bleomycin sulfate may develop pulmonary toxicity.

_____ 4. Antiemetics may be ordered to increase the client's appetite.

_____ 5. Stomatitis is a common side effect of vinorelbine sulfate.

Multiple Choice

Circle the best answer for each of the following questions. There is only one answer to each question.

1. Which of the following medications often causes toxicity to the hematopoietic system of the body?
   A. antimetabolites
   B. mitotic inhibitors
   C. alkylating agents
   D. antibiotics

2. The major form of toxicity that develops from the administration of doxorubicin HCl is
   A. cardiotoxicity
   B. neurotoxicity
   C. granulocytopenia
   D. ototoxicity

3. The major form of toxicity that develops from the administration of cyclophosphamide is

A. cardiotoxicity   C. hemorrhagic cystitis
B. neurotoxicity   D. ototoxicity

4. Clients receiving antineoplastic agents are at high risk for

A. diarrhea   C. infection
B. intractable pain   D. uric acid toxicity

5. You client has just completed his intravenous dose of methotrexate. You would expect to administer which of the following immediately?

A. mesna   C. triethylenethiophosphoramide
B. leucovorin calcium   D. streptozocin

6. The nurse understands that the maintenance intravenous fluid infused before and after intravenous methotrexate is

A. 10% dextrose/0.45% normal saline
B. lactated Ringer's solution
C. 0.9% sodium chloride
D. 5% dextrose and sodium bicarbonate

7. One adverse response to this medication, when given as an intravenous bolus to children, is rectal itching and burning.

A. dexamethasone   C. tamoxifen
B. toremifene citrate   D. polyestradiol phosphate

8. An important nursing assessment for the client receiving intravenous antineoplastic agents is

A. capillary blood glucose every four hours
B. urine specific gravity each void
C. continuous cardiac telemetry
D. urine protein every other void

9. Clients who receive methotrexate should have their uric acid levels monitored. Which of the following medications may be administered to inhibit formation of uric acid?

A. doxorubicin   C. allopurinol
B. colchicine   D. mesna

10. Clients with a Port-a-Cath receive medications through their port. What special precautions are needed?

A. use of a right-angle, non-coring needle
B. use of medical asepsis technique when accessing the port
C. change the access needle every 24 hours
D. flush port with heparin prior to accessing

Critical Thinking Exercises

1. Describe how cytotoxic agents are administered and disposed of after use.

_____

_____

_____

_____

2. Create a teaching plan for your client taking antineoplastic agents. Include nursing interventions and specify techniques for promoting client safety.

_____

_____

_____

_____

_____

3. Attend a local support group for cancer patients and their families. Describe your experience.

_____

_____

_____

_____

_____

4. Evaluate a local hospice program. Learn how they support terminally ill clients and their families.

_____

_____

_____

_____

_____

5. Obtain instructional materials from the American Cancer Society and prepare a presentation.

_____

_____

_____

_____

_____

CHAPTER 41 Agents Used in the Treatment of Eye Disorders

Objectives

After reading Chapter 41 of *Pharmacological Aspects of Nursing Care,* 7th edition, the student will be able to:

■ Discuss aqueous and vitreous humor.

■ Discuss the major types, therapeutic actions, and adverse effects of agents used for glaucoma.

■ Discuss the interactions between glaucoma agents and other medications.

■ Discuss agents that increase the outflow of aqueous humor from the eyes.

■ Discuss agents that decrease the production of aqueous humor.

■ Apply nursing interventions associated with the administration of glaucoma agents.

Matching

Match the following terms with their correct definitions.

_____ 1. narrow-angle glaucoma

_____ 2. carbonic-anhydrase inhibitors

_____ 3. open-angle glaucoma

_____ 4. osmotic diuretics

_____ 5. sympathomimetic agents

_____ 6. miotics

_____ 7. cholinesterase inhibitors

_____ 8. beta-adrenergic blockers

_____ 9. prostaglandin inhibitors

A. the iris occludes the anterior chamber structures of the eye and reduces outflow of aqueous humor

B. reduces the production of aqueous humor when applied topically

C. more toxic and longer acting; reserved for treatment of open-angle glaucoma when other treatments have failed

D. rapidly reduces production of aqueous humor by withdrawing fluid from the body

E. these drugs inhibit the action of carbonic anhydrase and are used in conjunction with topical agents

F. these medications inhibit the action of neurotransmitters and enzymes

G. no change in chamber angle, but degenerative changes impede the flow of aqueous humor

H. use of these medications may change the color of the iris

I. these medications stimulate adrenergic receptors in the eye

True or False

Place T or F on the line before each statement.

_____ 1. The most common adverse effect of pilocarpine is the reduction of visual acuity.

_____ 2. Pilocarpine is used to treat chronic open-angle glaucoma.

_____ 3. Antibiotic ointments are seldom used to treat eye infections because they are not sterile.

_____ 4. Clients receiving mydriatic agents should be aware of increased photosensitivity after administration.

_____ 5. Antibiotic eyedrops are usually effective on their own for eliminating infections from the eye.

Multiple Choice

Circle the best answer for each of the following questions. There is only one answer to each question.

1. Clients receiving idoxuridine may experience toxicity, as exhibited by

   A. irritation
   B. dry eye
   C. painless swelling
   D. decreased redness

2. Which clients are most likely to experience cardiovascular collapse or psychotic reaction when given tropicamide?

   A. young children
   B. the elderly
   C. clients with cardiac disease
   D. clients with renal disease

3. Which of the following medications may cause allergic contact dermatitis?

   A. proparacaine HCl
   B. dexamethasone
   C. phenylephrine HCl
   D. scopolamine HBr

4. Which of the following medications is used to loosen a cataract lens so that it may be surgically removed?

   A. tetracaine
   B. levocabastine HCl
   C. chymotrypsin
   D. hydroxyamphetamine HBr

5. Solutions of _____ may be used to precipitate and remove accumulated mucus in the eyes.

   A. peroxide
   B. silver nitrate
   C. calcium carbonate
   D. pilocarpine

6. Which of the following medications should not be used in clients receiving cholinesterase-inhibiting drugs, due to the possibility that respiratory depression may occur?

   A. atropine
   B. succinylcholine
   C. verapamil
   D. physostigmine salicylate

7. Systemic effects of miotics include

   A. reduced visual acuity
   B. poor illumination
   C. eye irritation
   D. gastrointestinal irritation

Critical Thinking Exercises

1. Create a presentation on the major types of medications used for the treatment of glaucoma, and describe their effects and contraindications.

   _____

   _____

   _____

   _____

   _____

2. Create a teaching plan for your client taking miotics, mydriatics, prostaglandin-inhibiting agents, cholinesterase-inhibiting agents, osmotic diuretics, and beta-adrenergic agents. Include interventions and ways to maintain client safety.

_____

_____

_____

_____

_____

3. Create a visual presentation, appropriate for client teaching, of the steps taken when administering eye drops.

_____

_____

_____

_____

_____

CHAPTER 42 Agents Used in the Treatment of Ear Disorders

Objectives

After reading Chapter 42 of *Pharmacological Aspects of Nursing Care,* 7th edition, the student will be able to:

■ Describe otic anti-infective agents, as well as their mechanisms of action, therapeutic effects, and side effects. Give an example of each.

■ Discuss the seven classifications of otic agents, as well as their mechanisms of action, therapeutic effects, and side effects. Give an example of each.

■ Discuss the differences between otitis media and the medications used to treat the condition.

■ Demonstrate the procedure for administering and applying otic agents.

Matching

Match the following terms with their correct definitions.

_____ 1. middle ear

_____ 2. inner ear

_____ 3. cerumen

_____ 4. pinna

_____ 5. cochlea

A. a waxy substance that helps to protect the ear canal

B. the outer, external ear

C. the sensory organ of hearing

D. the part of the ear where sound is conducted

E. contains the cochlea and semicircular canals

Multiple Choice

Circle the best answer for each of the following questions. There is only one answer to each question.

1. The first-line treatment for otitis media is

    A. systemic antimicrobials
    B. local antifungals
    C. ototopical agents
    D. wax emulsifiers

2. Otic medication must be administered in the ear by which method for children?

    A. pull the pinna up and back
    B. pull the pinna down and back
    C. either way is appropriate
    D. have the child sit with the affected ear facing down

3. The medication commonly used to treat an infection caused by Proteus mirabilis is

    A. gentamicin
    B. ciprofloxacin
    C. ofloxacin
    D. Cortisporin

4. Administration of which of the following medications has been shown to be effective against bacterial and fungal infections?

    A. acetic acid and hydrocortisone
    B. amoxicillin
    C. pramoxine and benzocaine
    D. carbamide peroxide

5. The treatment of otitis media often involves using this medication to reduce pain.

    A. hydrocortisone
    B. ofloxacin
    C. aluminum acetate
    D. acetic acid

6. Excess cerumen can alter auditory acuity and is treated with

    A. carbamide peroxide or Cortisporin
    B. pramoxine and benzocaine
    C. ear irrigations or carbamide peroxide
    D. acetic acid and ofloxacin

7. A mother brings her infant into the health clinic because "she has been fussy and pulling at her right ear for the past two days." How would you interpret this?

    A. The infant is probably experiencing colic.
    B. Infants often pull on their ears when they are experiencing anxiety.
    C. The mother is overreacting to the infant's actions.
    D. Infants often pull on an ear with otitis media to relieve the pressure in the ear.

Critical Thinking Exercises

1. Create a visual presentation of the seven classifications of otic agents, along with their mechanisms of action, therapeutic effects, and side effects.

    _____

    _____

    _____

    _____

2. Create a care plan for your client with an otitis media infection, including nursing interventions. Specify techniques for promoting pain relief and positive well-being.

    _____

    _____

    _____

    _____

3. Using Microsoft PowerPoint, create a presentation to illustrate how an infant's or child's ear anatomy differs from that of an adult.

    _____

    _____

    _____

    _____

CHAPTER 43 Agents Used in the Treatment of Skin Disorders

Objectives

After reading Chapter 43 of *Pharmacological Aspects of Nursing Care,* 7th edition, the student will be able to:

- Describe the structure of the skin and how the mechanisms of action of different medications help to relieve skin conditions.
- Discuss the therapeutic actions of keratolytics, emollients, local anesthetics, antifungals, and antiviral agents.
- Demonstrate the procedure for administering and applying topical agents.
- Describe therapeutic diets and the goals of nutritional changes that may improve skin conditions.

Matching

Match the following terms with their correct definitions.

_____ 1. emollients

_____ 2. keratolytic agents

_____ 3. antipruritics

_____ 4. sebaceous glands

_____ 5. stratum germinativum

_____ 6. antiviral agents

_____ 7. apocrine

A. new skin cells are formed in this layer of the skin

B. this medication is used to treat viral infections of the skin

C. connected to hair follicles, these are abundant on the head and face

D. these medications are oily substances that form an occlusive layer; applied to skin to prevent further loss of moisture

E. always connected to a hair follicle, these are not as widely dispersed as eccrine glands

F. these agents aid in removing excess keratin

G. these agents inhibit sensory nerve impulses and may contain antihistamines to decrease an immunological response

True or False

Place T or F on the line before each statement.

_____ 1. Emollients may be creams, oils, or lotions.

_____ 2. Keratolytics must be applied on an ongoing basis to maintain a state of remission.

_____ 3. The most common fungal infection is ringworm.

_____ 4. Herpes simplex I and II may be eradicated through the use of topical agents.

_____ 5. Anti-inflammatory agents are among the most effective treatments for irritation and allergic responses.

_____ 6. Scabies and lice infestation are caused by pediculosis corporis.

_____ 7. Diabetic foot ulcers often begin as fungal infections.

_____ 8. Minoxidil is commonly used as an antihypertensive agent.

_____ 9. An occlusive dressing should be applied after application of masoprocol.

_____ 10. Medication applied to a lesion is first applied to the center of the lesion and then spread outward to prevent contamination.

Multiple Choice

Circle the best answer for each of the following questions. There is only one answer to each question.

1. Grafts from the client's own skin are called

   A. autografts
   B. allografts
   C. xenografts
   D. heterografts

2. This medication is a solution that must be kept saturated to prevent the burning of tissue.

   A. masoprocol
   B. sutilains
   C. collagenase
   D. silver nitrate

3. The most significant adverse effect of lindane administration is

   A. eczema
   B. seizures in children
   C. central nervous system (CNS) toxicity
   D. renal failure

4. Acyclovir is administered for the treatment of which of the following conditions?

   A. dermatitis
   B. glitazones
   C. herpes simplex
   D. fungal infections

5. The treatment of acne vulgaris may consist of

   A. topical antibacterial agents
   B. acetaminophen
   C. anti-inflammatories
   D. acyclovir

6. Fluorouracil is a topical agent used to treat

   A. sunburn
   B. actinic keratosis
   C. burns
   D. pediculosis

7. Clients with extensive burns are at high risk for which of the following conditions?

   A. edema
   B. infection
   C. future burns
   D. cardiac dysrhythmias

8. After applying this medication topically, the urine may turn dark red in color.

   A. silver sulfadiazine
   B. sutilains
   C. nitrofurazone
   D. haloprogin

Critical Thinking Exercises

1. Create a visual presentation of the functions of the human skin.

   _____

   _____

   _____

   _____

   _____

2. Create a care plan for your client with a chronic skin condition (such as psoriasis or cystic acne vulgaris), including nursing interventions. Specify techniques for promoting self-esteem and positive well-being.

_____

_____

_____

_____

_____

3. Using at least one Internet Web site, research ways to identify skin conditions occurring on dark-skinned individuals.

_____

_____

_____

_____

_____

ANSWER KEY

Chapter 1

Matching
1. C
2. D
3. E
4. B
5. A
6. B
7. E
8. A
9. D
10. C
11. C
12. B
13. E
14. A
15. D

True or False
1. F
2. T
3. T
4. T
5. F
6. F
7. T
8. F
9. T
10. T

Multiple Choice
1. A
2. B
3. D
4. C
5. C
6. C
7. A
8. B
9. C
10. A

Chapter 2

Matching
1. C
2. A
3. D
4. B
5. E
6. B
7. D
8. C
9. A
10. G
11. H
12. E
13. F
14. I

True or False
1. T
2. F
3. F
4. T
5. T
6. F
7. T
8. F
9. F
10. F
11. T
12. T
13. T
14. F
15. T

Multiple Choice
1. C
2. B
3. D
4. C
5. B
6. A
7. C
8. A
9. D
10. B
11. B
12. A

Chapter 3

Matching
1. D
2. A
3. C
4. B
5. E

True or False
1. T
2. T
3. F
4. T
5. T
6. F
7. T
8. T
9. F
10. T

Multiple Choice
1. B
2. A
3. D
4. C
5. C
6. B
7. D
8. C

Chapter 4

Matching
1. B
2. D
3. C
4. A

True or False
1. T
2. T
3. F
4. T
5. T

Practice Problems
1. 0.5 mL
2. 1 tablet
3. 1.25 mL
4. 8 mL
5. 250 mL
6. 4 capsules
7. ½ tablet
8. 2 tablets
9. 12 mL
10. 10 mg; 5 mg/dose
11. ½ mL
12. 50 gtt/min
13. 12.5 mL/hour
14. 8 hours
15. 200 mL/hour

Chapter 5

Matching
1. B
2. C
3. A
4. D

True or False
1. F
2. F
3. T
4. T

Multiple Choice
1. A
2. B
3. C
4. B
5. D
6. A
7. D
8. A
9. D

Chapter 6

Matching
1. B
2. C
3. D
4. A
5. A
6. B
7. C
8. D
9. E

True or False
1. T
2. F
3. F
4. T

Multiple Choice
1. B
2. B
3. C
4. B
5. D
6. A
7. B
8. C

Chapter 7

Matching
1. E
2. C
3. F
4. B
5. D
6. A
7. A
8. B
9. E
10. C
11. D

True or False
1. T
2. T
3. T
4. T
5. T
6. F
7. T
8. F
9. T
10. T

Multiple Choice
1. B
2. A
3. D
4. B
5. C
6. D
7. C
8. C
9. D
10. C

Chapter 8

Matching
1. C
2. B
3. A
4. D
5. E

True or False
1. T
2. T
3. T
4. F
5. T

Multiple Choice
1. A
2. B
3. A
4. C
5. A
6. A
7. D
8. C
9. C
10. A

Chapter 9

Matching
1. D
2. B
3. E
4. A
5. C

True or False
1. F
2. T
3. T
4. T
5. F
6. T
7. T
8. T

Multiple Choice
1. D
2. A
3. C
4. B
5. B
6. C
7. D
8. A
9. B

Chapter 10

Matching
1. D
2. C
3. B
4. A
5. E
6. F

True or False
1. F
2. T
3. T
4. T
5. F
6. F

Multiple Choice
1. A
2. B
3. B
4. C
5. A
6. C
7. D
8. A
9. A
10. D

Chapter 11

Matching
1. D
2. B
3. C
4. E
5. A

True or False
1. T
2. F
3. F
4. F
5. F

Multiple Choice
1. D
2. C
3. B
4. D
5. C
6. B
7. A
8. C
9. B
10. D

Chapter 12

Matching
1. G
2. A
3. C
4. E
5. F
6. B
7. D

True or False
1. F
2. F
3. F
4. T
5. T
6. T
7. F
8. T

Multiple Choice
1. B
2. D
3. A
4. B
5. B
6. C
7. D
8. C

Chapter 13

Matching
1. B
2. D
3. A
4. E
5. C
6. F

True or False
1. T
2. T
3. F
4. F
5. F

Multiple Choice
1. B
2. B
3. D
4. B
5. B
6. B
7. A

Chapter 14

Matching
1. C
2. E
3. A
4. B
5. D
6. F

True or False
1. T
2. F
3. T
4. F
5. F
6. T
7. T

Multiple Choice
1. C
2. A
3. C
4. D
5. C
6. B
7. A
8. C

Chapter 15

Matching
1. D
2. A
3. C

True or False
1. F
2. F
3. T

Multiple Choice
1. D
2. C
3. A
4. D
5. B
6. A
7. A

Chapter 16

Matching
1. E
2. D
3. A
4. F
5. G
6. H
7. B
8. C

True or False
1. T
2. T
3. T
4. F
5. F
6. T

Multiple Choice
1. C
2. A
3. B
4. A
5. B
6. B
7. C
8. D

Chapter 17

Matching
1. F
2. B
3. D
4. E
5. H
6. G
7. J
8. I
9. A
10. C

True or False
1. F
2. F
3. F
4. T
5. T

Multiple Choice
1. A
2. D
3. D
4. C
5. A
6. B
7. A
8. D
9. C
10. D
11. B
12. A

Chapter 18

Matching
1. D
2. C
3. B
4. A

True or False
1. F
2. T
3. F
4. T
5. F
6. T

Multiple Choice
1. A
2. D
3. C
4. C
5. C
6. B
7. D
8. B
9. A
10. B

Chapter 19

Matching
1. D
2. A
3. C
4. B
5. E

True or False
1. F
2. F
3. F
4. T
5. F

Multiple Choice
1. B
2. C
3. A
4. A
5. A
6. B
7. D
8. C
9. B
10. C
11. B

Chapter 20

Matching
1. A
2. E
3. D
4. C
5. B

True or False
1. T
2. T
3. T
4. T
5. F

Multiple Choice
1. C
2. D
3. A
4. A
5. C
6. D
7. A
8. B
9. D
10. B
11. C
12. A

Chapter 21

Matching
1. D
2. E
3. C
4. B
5. A

True or False
1. T
2. F
3. F
4. F
5. T

Multiple Choice
1. C
2. A
3. C
4. A
5. A
6. C
7. D

Chapter 22

Matching
1. B
2. D
3. C
4. E
5. A

True or False
1. T
2. T
3. F
4. F

Multiple Choice
1. C
2. D
3. A
4. C
5. B
6. D
7. C
8. D
9. A
10. B

Chapter 23

Matching
1. F
2. H
3. I
4. A
5. D
6. G
7. B
8. C
9. E

True or False
1. T
2. T
3. F
4. F
5. T

Multiple Choice
1. A
2. B
3. C
4. B
5. C
6. A
7. D
8. C
9. A
10. D
11. B
12. B

Chapter 24

Matching
1. B
2. E
3. D
4. C
5. A

True or False
1. F
2. F
3. F
4. F

Multiple Choice
1. C
2. A
3. A
4. C
5. D

Chapter 25

Matching
1. C
2. A
3. D
4. E
5. F
6. B

True or False
1. F
2. F
3. T
4. F
5. T
6. T

Multiple Choice
1. B
2. A
3. D
4. C
5. D
6. C
7. A
8. B
9. A
10. A

Chapter 26

Matching
1. E
2. D
3. A
4. C
5. B
6. G
7. F

True or False
1. T
2. F
3. T
4. F
5. T

Multiple Choice
1. A
2. A
3. C
4. B
5. B
6. C
7. C

Chapter 27

Matching
1. C
2. B
3. D
4. A

True or False
1. F
2. T
3. F
4. T
5. F
6. T
7. T
8. F
9. F
10. T

Multiple Choice
1. A
2. C
3. C
4. D
5. E
6. D
7. C
8. D
9. A
10. B

Chapter 28

Matching
1. C
2. E
3. A
4. B
5. G
6. F
7. D
8. H

Multiple Choice
1. B
2. C
3. C
4. D
5. A
6. B
7. A

Chapter 29

Matching
1. C
2. D
3. G
4. A
5. F
6. B
7. H
8. E

True or False
1. F
2. F
3. T
4. F
5. F
6. T

Multiple Choice
1. C
2. A
3. C

Chapter 30

Matching
1. A
2. F
3. D
4. C
5. B
6. E
7. H
8. G

True or False
1. F
2. F
3. T
4. T
5. F
6. F

Multiple Choice
1. C
2. C
3. B
4. A
5. A
6. C
7. A
8. C

Chapter 31

Matching
1. C
2. E
3. B
4. A
5. F
6. D

True or False
1. F
2. F
3. T
4. F
5. F
6. F
7. F
8. F

Multiple Choice
1. C
2. B
3. D
4. D
5. C
6. A
7. C
8. B

Chapter 32

Matching
1. A
2. B
3. D
4. F
5. G
6. C
7. E
8. H

True or False
1. F
2. F
3. F
4. F
5. F
6. T
7. T
8. F

Multiple Choice
1. D
2. A
3. C
4. C
5. B
6. D
7. A
8. A
9. A
10. D

Chapter 33

Matching
1. D
2. E
3. C
4. A
5. B

True or False
1. F
2. F
3. T
4. T
5. F

Multiple Choice
1. A
2. C
3. B
4. A
5. C
6. C
7. B
8. D
9. B
10. B
11. D

Chapter 34

Matching
1. D
2. A
3. B
4. C
5. E
6. I
7. H
8. F
9. J
10. G

True or False
1. T
2. T
3. T
4. F
5. F
6. F
7. T
8. F
9. T
10. T

Multiple Choice
1. E
2. D
3. D
4. C
5. C
6. A
7. A
8. D
9. B
10. B

Chapter 35

Matching
1. D
2. G
3. E
4. H
5. A
6. B
7. F
8. C

True or False
1. F
2. T
3. F
4. T
5. T

Multiple Choice
1. B
2. A
3. A
4. C
5. C
6. C
7. D
8. D
9. D
10. A

Chapter 36

Matching
1. B
2. G
3. F
4. C
5. D
6. H
7. A
8. E
9. I

True or False
1. T
2. T
3. F
4. T
5. T

Multiple Choice
1. C
2. A
3. C
4. C
5. A
6. B
7. D
8. D
9. C
10. B

Chapter 37

Matching
1. C
2. E
3. G
4. F
5. A
6. B
7. D

True or False
1. F
2. T
3. T
4. T
5. F

Multiple Choice
1. C
2. A
3. C
4. B
5. D
6. D
7. B
8. A
9. B

Chapter 38

Matching
1. C
2. A
3. B

True or False
1. T
2. F
3. T
4. F

Multiple Choice
1. C
2. D
3. B
4. A
5. D

Chapter 39

Matching
1. D
2. C
3. B
4. A

Multiple Choice
1. A
2. C
3. D
4. D
5. B
6. A
7. D
8. D

Chapter 40

Matching
1. D
2. A
3. F
4. C
5. B
6. E

True or False
1. T
2. F
3. T
4. T
5. F

Multiple Choice
1. C
2. A
3. C
4. C
5. B
6. D
7. A
8. B
9. C
10. A

Chapter 41

Matching
1. A
2. E
3. G
4. D
5. I
6. F
7. C
8. B
9. H

True or False
1. T
2. T
3. F
4. T
5. F

Multiple Choice
1. A
2. A
3. A
4. C
5. B
6. B
7. D

Chapter 42

Matching
1. D
2. E
3. A
4. B
5. C

Multiple Choice
1. A
2. B
3. B
4. A
5. A
6. C
7. D

Chapter 43

Matching
1. D
2. F
3. G
4. C
5. A
6. B
7. E

True or False
1. T
2. F
3. T
4. F
5. T
6. F
7. F
8. T
9. F
10. T

Multiple Choice
1. A
2. D
3. B
4. C
5. A
6. B
7. B
8. C